CONTENTS

Introduction

Do you and your partner have a complicated relationship with food?
Do you both think that you are eating healthy and your weight is instead growing up?
Are you making enough effort but couldn't get your diet on track?
Do you wish for a miracle diet that could just wipe your health problems?
If any of the answer of the above questions is yes, then look no further and get started with the Keto diet.

Keto diet is the trendiest diet of 2019 that has charmed celebrities, fitness freaks, dieticians, and health professionals.Even tech workers in Silicon Valley are a fan of the Keto diet. Keto diet is not just limited to lose fats; it plays a major role in shedding excess body fat and maintain a healthy weight. A Keto diet does this all by entering the body into Ketosis with the help of very low carb and high-fat food. And as a result, Keto food switches your energy source from carbs (glucose) to fats (Ketone).

In Keto diet, you are not just eating to eat; you are putting something in your mouth that will create a positive impact on your health. I know this means that you will have to leave your favorite pasta, pizza, and potatoes, but once your taste buds become habitual to delicious Keto foods, you will not feel that your food is holding you back.

So, do you want to give a shot to Keto diet?
Read on and find out what Keto diet is and how it can change your and your significant other life. You won't believe the places you lose weight with Keto meal planning for more than a week.

Chapter 1 Keto Diet Basics

There are varieties of low carb diet, which is a diet high in fats, moderate in protein, and low in carbs. But Keto diet is a special low carb type. But how much low? Keto diet contains very low or no-carb in food. The number of carbs varies depending on the activity level and insulin tolerance. Keto food has 20g or less net carbs. Net carbs is a difference between total carbs and fiber. So, when you are shopping for your meal, just look at the net carbs of the ingredients and purchases accordingly.

This doesn't mean Keto diet is Paleo, Atkins, or high protein. The difference in macronutrient on Keto make its unique and difference from other low-carb diets. You need to focus on the macronutrients for planning a Keto diet, rather than counting calories. Carb, protein and fat are macronutrients, and in Keto diet, there are 70 percent or more 'good' fats, 20 to 25 percent protein and maximum 10 percent carbohydrates.

What is Keto Diet, And How Does it Work?

Keto diet aims to make the body reach a state called Ketosis. Ketosis is a metabolic state in which the body burns fats instead of carbs as a fuel. This process of burning fats is very effective for weight loss, mental clarity, and boost energy.

Our body normally uses carbohydrates and burn them for energy. When you are on a Keto diet which restricts carbs, the body will first burn all the stored carbs for energy and then switch to store fats. As a result, fats are breakdown into molecules called ketones, which are then used as fuel. There is nothing dangerous about Ketosis, as it is a normal process. It's just that Keto lifestyle keeps your body constantly in that state.

The body normally takes three days to enter Ketosis after starting a Keto diet. However, there are many ways to speed up this process, such as:

1- Reducing carb consumption significantly in your food. Aim to eat 20-grams carbs or less per day.

2- Increase the intake of healthy fats. And for this, use coconut oil, olive oil, avocado oil, flaxseed oil or MCT oil generously in your foods.

3- Maintain a high protein intake. Remember that Keto is not a high-protein diet, so don't go overboard with it because excess protein is stored as glucose in the body that make it harder for you to go in Ketosis.

4- Increase physical activity and exercise more. The more you exercise, the more energy you will generate by depleting carbs reserves and then fat stores in the body.

5- Do fasting between meals with a window of 12 to 16 hours. You can also go for a longer period of fasting like 24 to 48 hours.

What to Eat and What to Avoid?

Here are healthy foods that you can eat on a Keto diet.

1- Meat: All unprocessed, organic and grass-fed meats – chicken, beef, steak, lamb, ham, pork, bacon, turkey and sausage

2- Fish and seafood: Eat wild-caught fishes and seafood – salmon, tuna, cod, snapper, trout, halibut, catfish, shrimps, crabs, oysters, scallops and mussels

3- Eggs: Organic and pastured eggs

4- Fats: High-fat oil, sauces, and dairy items – high-fat cheese, high fat yogurt, heavy cream, coconut milk, almond milk, avocado oil, coconut oil, butter, almond butter, clarified butter, mayonnaise, and high-fat sauces

5- Nuts: Have nuts in moderate amount – peanut, almond, walnuts, hazelnuts, macadamia nuts, and pecans
6- Vegetables: Vegetables that grow about the ground and are low in carbs – avocado, zucchini, cauliflower, broccoli, cabbage, olives, peppers, onion, tomato, cucumber, mushroom, asparagus, green beans, spinach, kale and lettuce
7- Berries: Berries that have a low glycemic index – raspberries, blueberries, blackberries, and strawberries (moderately)
8- Drinks: Keep yourself hydrated by drinking plenty of water, with ice or sliced cucumbers and limes or lemon. You are also allowed to have coffee (unsweetened), tea such as herbal, mint, green, or black tea (without added sugar). Bone broth is also a great beverage to sip on Keto. You have alcohol like dry red or white wine, champagne, cocktails, whiskey, and brandy (without sugar) on special occasions in moderate amount.
9- Sweeteners: Use sweeteners sparingly – stevia, erythritol, and zero-calorie sweetener
Following are the list of food that you must avoid on the keto diet.
1- Grains and starches: All rice, wheat, buckwheat, oats, quinoa, legumes, beans, lentil, millets, chickpeas, amaranth, and sprouted grain
2- Vegetables: All root and high carb vegetables – regular potato, sweet potato, carrot, turnip, yam, beetroot, parsnip, peas
3- Fruits: High sugar and glycemic index fruits – apple, melon, banana, oranges, peaches, plum, mangoes, pears, cherries, grapes, pineapple
4- Grain products: All food items made from grains and flour – bread, cake, buns, pasta, cookies, cereal, crackers, pizza, bagel, corn, oatmeal
5- Sweets: All artificial and high sugar sweeteners and sweets – honey, white sugar, cane sugar, maple syrup, agave nectar, corn syrup, candy, tarts, pies, pastries, pudding, custard
6- Oils: Sesame oil, sunflower oil, canola oil, and soybean oil
7- Drinks: High carb juices and smoothies, soda, beer, sweet wines, sweet alcoholic drinks, tea, and coffee
8- Dairy: All low-fat dairy items such as low-fat cheeses like skim mozzarella cheese, low-fat yogurt, cream cheese, skim milk
9- Sweetened sauces, dips and salad dressing

Benefits of Keto Diet

The major reason for the popularly of the Keto diet is its innumerable benefits.
Weight loss
Control cravings
Improve digestion
Less bloating and gas
Reduce acne
Better sleep
Rise in energy level
Increased memory and clarity
Diminishes depression and anxiety
Fewer migraines
Improve arthritis and pain
Sharpen brain
Stable vision

Inflammation markers fall
A healthier liver
Boost heart health
Less heartburn
Improve brain functioning
Reduce the risk of tumors and seizures
Less risk for gall stones
Aid recovery from brain injuries
Maintain uric acid levels
Increase fertility in women
Curb diabetes
Treat several types of cancer, polycystic ovarian syndrome (PCOS), neurological disorders and metabolic syndromes and diseases

Keto Tips and Inspiration for Two

Starting a Keto diet can be difficult, and if you are doing it alone, you may face lots of difficulties, then the results won't turn out as it should be. However, your significant other can make your Keto transition way to easier. Couples who diet together are more likely to meet their health goals. Your partner can be the listener of your all Keto experiences, an accountability partners who really understand what you are going through.

But ... is your significant other bickering so much? Or, annoying than usual? Is stress getting thicker? And, you both are finding it hard to stick to your very simple plan. So, is it not worth doing it together?

Of course not! This is just a phase because your body is in adapting mode, and once the transition is done, you both will get back to your true self. Until then, have patience and believe in your teamwork potential. You both will get through this phase.

Following are some tips for you and your lover to make your Keto lifestyle changes together as easy as possible.

Focus on developing healthy eating habits. Set a time in a well to prepare your grocery list together and then organize meals for the week or month ahead.

Discuss what you want to achieve with Keto diet. Is it weight loss or just to have more energy? Then talk about how you would achieve your goal and what should you do together about it. You don't need to have same Keto goals, but you need to be clear about them from the start so that you can encourage each other throughout your Keto experience.

Don't be your partner's drill sergeant. The bossy attitude is old. Instead, you both need to be personally accountable for what you do. Make an exercise chart together or schedule physical activity time on your shared online calendar. Invite your partner for exercise or gym, but don't push more than that.

A healthy competition between you and your partner can be motivating and fun. However, too much teasing can take this the wrong way. So be supportive as much as possible, be considerate to your partner progress and keep the funny comments to yourself.

You Both Can And Will Do This Together!

Chapter 2 Breakfast (Brunch) Recipes

Cheese Crusted Omelet

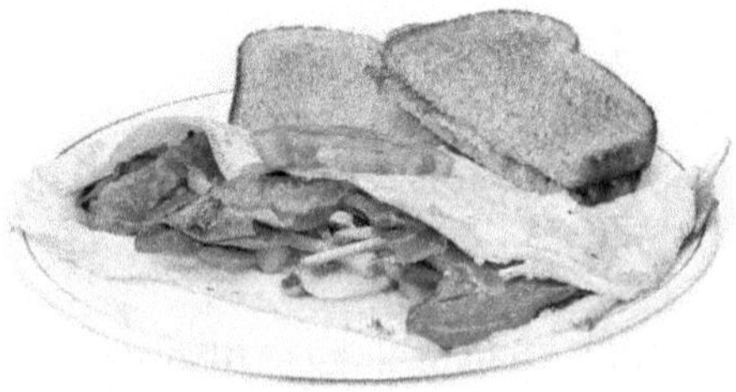

Prep time: 5 minutes, Cooking time: 16 minutes, Servings: 2

Ingredients

For Omelet

- Eggs - 4
- Salt - ½ tsp
- Ground black pepper - ½ tsp
- Heavy whipping cream - 4 tbsp
- Butter or coconut oil - 2 tbsp
- Shredded cheddar cheese - 6 oz

For Filling

- Mushrooms, sliced - 4
- Baby spinach - 1 oz
- Cherry tomatoes, sliced - 4
- Deli turkey - 2 oz
- Cream cheese - 4 tbsp
- Dried oregano - 2 tsp

Instructions

1. Prepare omelet and for this, crack eggs in a bowl, season with salt and black pepper, then add cream and whisk until combined.
2. Place a non-stick skillet pan over medium heat, add 1 tablespoon butter and when it melts, spread half of the cheese in the pan and fry until bubbly.
3. Then turn heat to the lower level, pour in half of the egg mixture over the melted cheese and cook for 2 minutes or until set, don't stir.
4. Top one half of omelet with half of each ingredient for filling and continue frying for 1 to 2 minutes or until set.
5. Then turn the other half of omelet over the filling, cook for 2 minutes and slide onto a plate.
6. Cook another omelet in the same manner by using the remaining ingredients.
7. Serve straight away.

Nutritional facts

Calories: 789; Fat: 66g; Saturated fat: 39g; Net Carbohydrate: 8g; Protein: 41g; Fiber: 2g;

Frittata Muffin Cups

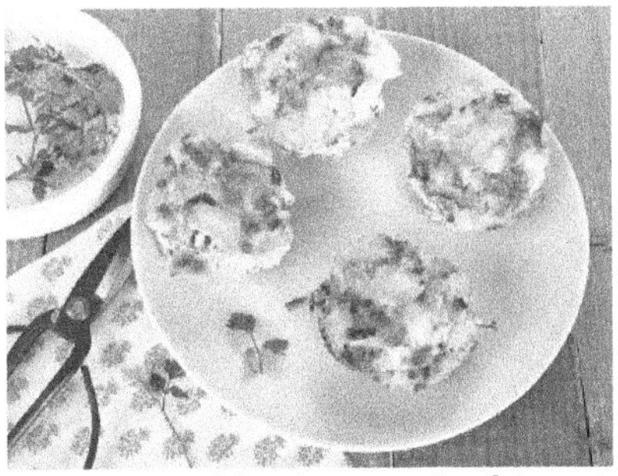

Prep time: 10 minutes, Cooking time: 18 minutes, Servings: 2

Ingredients

- Bacon, cooked and chopped – 3 oz
- Eggs – 4
- Half-and-half –¼ cup
- Salt – 1/8 tsp
- Ground black pepper – 1/4 tsp
- Dried parsley – 1 tsp
- Shredded cheddar cheese – ¼ cup
- Butter – ½ tbsp

Instructions

1. Set oven to 375 ° F and let preheat.
2. Crack eggs in a large bowl, add half-and-half and whisk until combined.
3. Add bacon and cheese, season with salt, black pepper, and parsley and fold until well mixed.
4. Take four silicon muffin cups, grease them with butter, and evenly fill with prepared muffin batter.
5. Place muffin cups into the oven and bake for 15 to 18 minutes or until the top is nicely golden brown and inserted toothpick into each muffin comes out clean.
6. When done, let muffin cool in cups for 1 minute, then turn them out and serve.

Nutritional facts

Calories: 112.4; Fat: 9.6g; Saturated fat: 3g; Net Carbohydrate: 0.9g; Protein: 8g; Fiber: 0.04g;

Frittata with Spinach

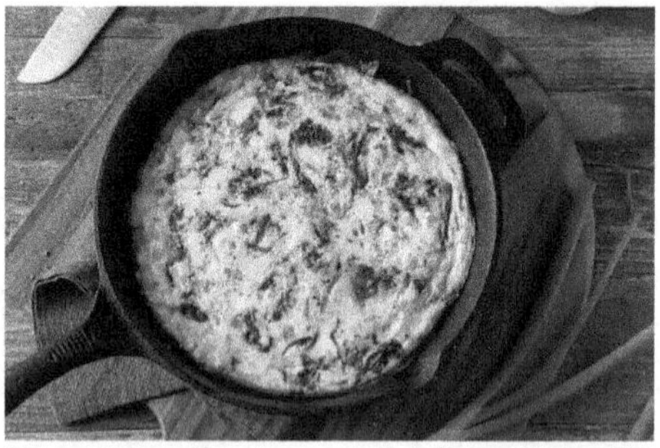

Prep time: 5 minutes, Cooking time: 38 minutes, Servings: 2

Ingredients

- Diced chorizo - 2½ oz.
- Butter - 1 tbsp
- Fresh spinach - 4 oz.
- Eggs - 4
- Heavy whipping cream - ½ cup
- Shredded cheddar cheese - 2½ oz.
- Salt - ½ tsp
- Ground black pepper - ½ tsp

Instructions

1. Set oven to 350 ° F and let preheat.
2. Meanwhile, place a skillet pan over medium heat, add butter and chorizo and cook for 3 to 5 minutes or until crispy.
3. Add spinach, continue cooking for 3 minutes or until leaves wilts, then remove the pan from heat and set aside until required.
4. Crack eggs in a bowl, add cream, whisk until smooth and then evenly divide into a square greased baking dish.
5. Top with bacon mixture, sprinkle with cheese and then place the baking dish into the oven.
6. Bake frittata for 25 to 30 minutes or until the top is nicely golden brown and the frittata is cooked through.
7. Divide frittata into two portions and serve.

Nutritional facts

Calories: 661; Fat: 59g; Saturated fat: 36g; Net Carbohydrate: 4g; Protein: 27g; Fiber: 1g;

French Pancakes

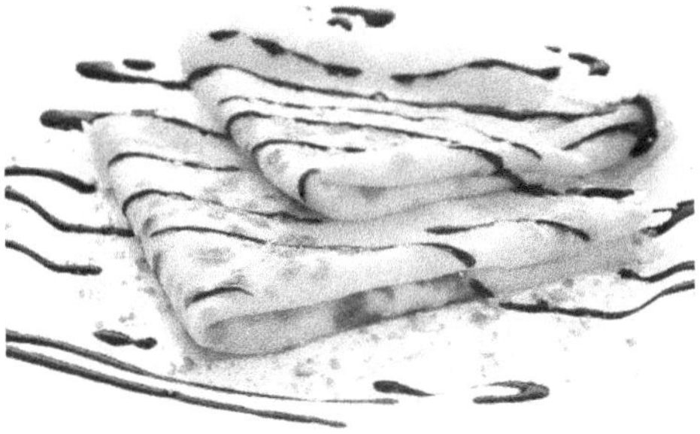

Prep time: 15 minutes, Cooking time: 14 minutes, Servings: 2

Ingredients

- Eggs – 4
- Salt – 1/8 tsp
- Heavy whipping cream – 1 cup
- Water – ¼ cup
- Psyllium husk powder, grounded – 1 tbsp
- Butter – 1½ oz.

Instructions

1. Crack eggs in a bowl, season with salt, add cream and water and whisk until smooth.
2. Then gradually whisk in husk power until smooth batter comes together and let rest for 10 minutes at room temperature.
3. After 10 minutes, place a skillet pan over medium-high heat, add butter and when it melts, add half of the pancake batter and spread evenly.
4. Cook pancake for 3 to 4 minutes or until the top is almost dry, then flip the pancake and continue cooking for 2 to 3 minutes or until nicely golden brown.
5. When done, slide pancake to a plate and use the remaining batter for cooking another pancake.
6. Serve straight away.

Nutritional facts

Calories: 688; Fat: 68g; Saturated fat: 49g; Net Carbohydrate: 1g; Protein: 15g; Fiber: 3g;

Cheesy Bacon Cornbread Waffles

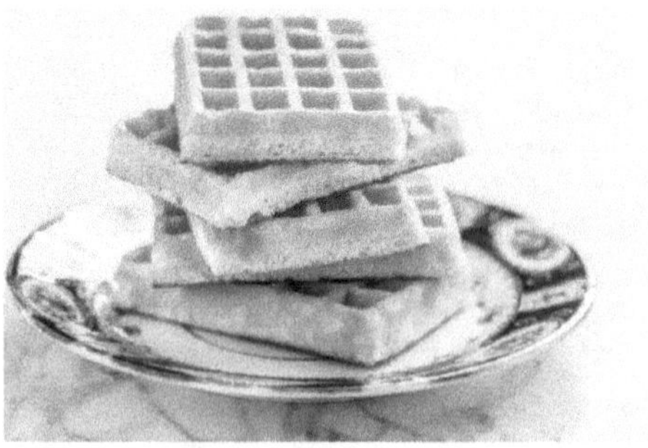

Prep time: 10 minutes, Cooking time: 5 minutes, Servings: 2

Ingredients

- Cooked bacon, chopped – 1 oz.
- Medium scallion, chopped – ½
- Coconut flour – 1 tbsp
- Oat fiber – 1 ½ tbsp
- Whey protein powder – 1 ½ tbsp
- Baking powder – 2/5 tsp
- Salt – 1/10 tsp
- Shredded cheddar cheese – 2 tbsp
- Butter, melted – 1 oz.
- Coconut oil, melted – 1 ½ tbsp
- Water – 1 tbsp
- Egg – 1

Instructions

1. Plugin and switch waffle iron and preheat as per manufacturer directions.
2. Meanwhile, place bacon in a bowl, add scallion, flour, oat, protein powder, baking powder, salt and cheese and stir until mixed.
3. Then remaining ingredients and whisk until smooth batter comes together.
4. Spoon half of the prepared batter into the waffle iron and cook until nicely golden brown and crispy.
5. Cook another waffle in the same manner by using the remaining batter.
6. Serve straight away.

Nutritional facts

Calories: 327; Fat: 31g; Saturated fat: 14g; Net Carbohydrate: 1g; Protein: 11g; Fiber: 5g;

French toast

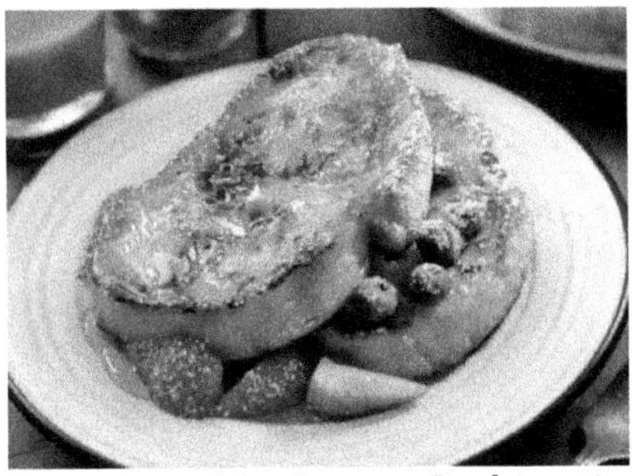

Prep time: 25 minutes, Cooking time: 10 minutes, Servings: 2

Ingredients

For Mug bread

- Almond flour - 2 tbsp
- Coconut flour - 2 tbsp
- Baking powder - 1½ tsp
- Salt - 1/16 tsp
- Butter - 1 tsp
- Eggs - 2
- Heavy whipping cream - 2 tbsp

For Batter

- Eggs - 2
- Salt - 1/16 tsp
- Ground cinnamon - ½ tsp
- Heavy whipping cream - 2 tbsp
- Butter - 2 tbsp

Instructions

1. Take a heatproof mug, grease it with butter, then add all flours, baking powder, and salt and stir until mixed.
2. Crack eggs in it, then add cream and whisk until smooth batter comes together.
3. Place the mug into the microwave and cook for 2 minutes at high heat setting or until bread is cooked through, check bread by inserting a toothpick into the center, and it should come out clean.
4. When done, remove mug from oven and let cool for 15 minutes.
5. Then take out bread and slice in half.
6. Prepare batter and for this, crack eggs in a bowl, add salt, cinnamon, and cream and whisk until smooth.
7. Pour this mixture over the bread slices and let soak completely, turning slices a few times.
8. Then place a skillet pan over medium heat, add butter and when it melts, add bread slices and cook for 3 to 4 minutes per side or until nicely golden brown and crispy.
9. Serve straight away with berries.

Nutritional facts

Calories: 416; Fat: 37g; Saturated fat: 17g; Net Carbohydrate: 4g; Protein: 15g; Fiber: 4g;

Mexican Scrambled Eggs

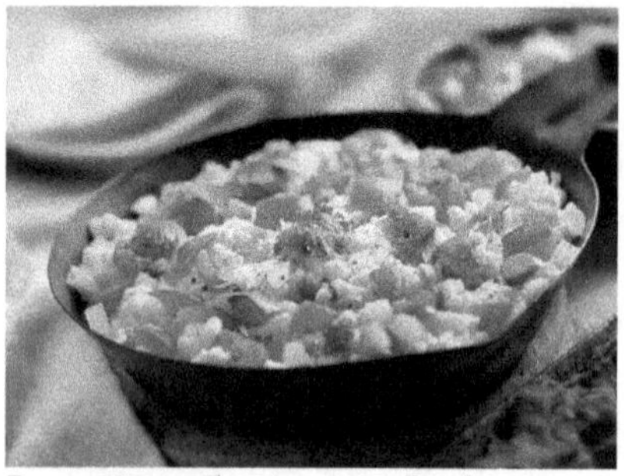

Prep time: 5 minutes, Cooking time: 5 minutes, Servings: 2

Ingredients

- Salt – ½ tsp
- Eggs – 3
- Scallion, chopped – ½
- Medium tomato, chopped – ½
- Pickled jalapeño, chopped – 1
- Shredded cheddar cheese – 1½ oz.
- Butter – 1 tbsp
- Salt – ½ tsp
- Ground black pepper – ½ tsp

Instructions

1. Place a large skillet pan over medium-high heat, add butter and when it melts, add scallion, tomato, and jalapeno and cook for 3 minutes or until beginning to soften.
2. Meanwhile, crack eggs in a bowl and whisk until beaten.
3. Pour the egg mixture into the pan, scramble eggs for 2 minutes, then sprinkle cheese on top and season with salt and black pepper.
4. Serve straight away.

Nutritional facts

Calories: 229; Fat: 12g; Saturated fat: 4g; Net Carbohydrate: 2g; Protein: 14g; Fiber: 1g;

Coconut Porridge

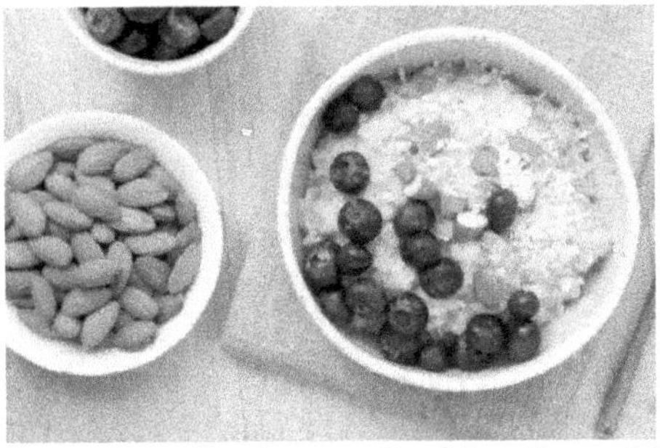

Prep time: 5 minutes, Cooking time: 10 minutes, Servings: 2

Ingredients

- Eggs, beaten – 2
- Coconut flour – 2 tbsp
- Salt – 1/8 teaspoon
- Psyllium husk powder grounded – 1/8 teaspoon
- Butter – 2 oz.
- Coconut cream – 8 tbsp

Instructions

1. Crack eggs in a bowl, add flour, salt, and Psyllium husk and whisk until combined.
2. Place a saucepan over low heat, add butter and when it melts, whisk in coconut cream.
3. Then slowly whisk in egg mixture until a smooth and creamy mixture comes together.
4. Divide porridge evenly between two bowls and serve with berries.

Nutritional facts

Calories: 486; Fat: 49g; Saturated fat: 28g; Net Carbohydrate: 4g; Protein: 9g; Fiber: 5g;

Cauliflower Hash Browns

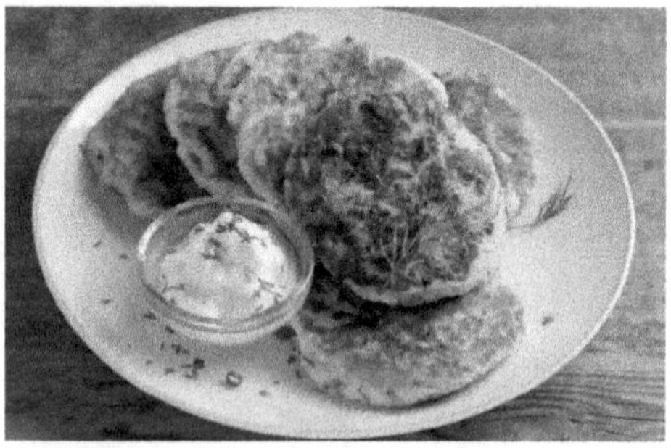

Prep time: 10 minutes, Cooking time: 30 minutes, Servings: 2

Ingredients

- Salt – ½ tsp
- Cauliflower, grated – ½ lb
- Eggs – 2
- White onion, grated – ¼
- Salt – ½ tsp
- Ground black pepper – ¼ tsp
- Butter, for frying – 2 oz.

Instructions

1. Place grated cauliflower in a bowl, add remaining ingredients and stir until mixed, let the mixture rest for 10 minutes.
2. Then place a skillet pan over medium heat, add butter and when it melts, lower the heat and place scoops of the cauliflower mixture.
3. Flatten each mixture into 3 to 4-inch patties and fry for 4 to 5 minutes per side or until nicely golden brown and cooked.
4. Serve straight away.

Nutritional facts

Calories: 282; Fat: 26g; Saturated fat: 9g; Net Carbohydrate: 5g; Protein: 7g; Fiber: 3g;

Chia Pudding

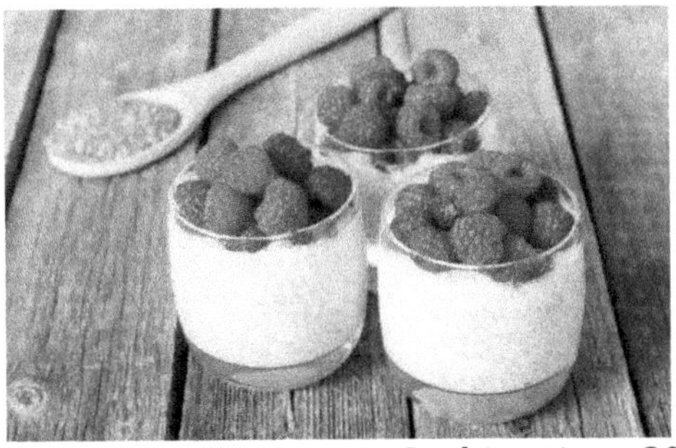

Prep time: 10 minutes, Cooking time: 20 minutes, Servings: 2

Ingredients

- Coconut milk, unsweetened – 2 cups
- Vanilla extract, unsweetened – 1 tsp
- Chia seeds – 4 tbsp

Instructions

1. Place all the ingredients in a bowl and blend until smooth mixture comes together.
2. Cover the bowl, then place in refrigerator and let rest for 4 hours or overnight.
3. Evenly divide pudding between two bowls and serve with berries.

Nutritional facts

Calories: 568; Fat: 12g; Saturated fat: 25g; Net Carbohydrate: 8g; Protein: 9g; Fiber: 8g;

Spinach and Avocado Smoothie

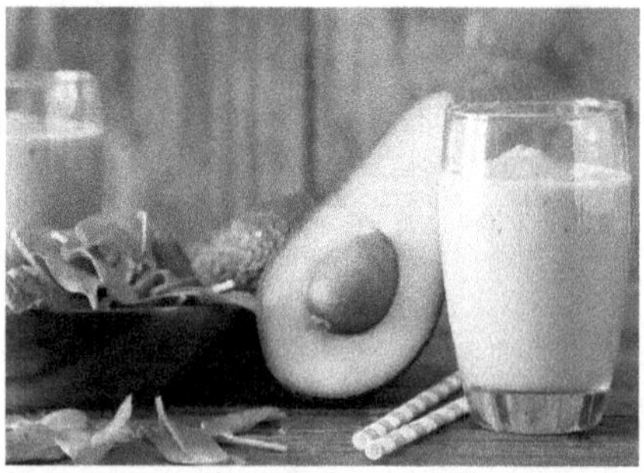

Prep time: 5 minutes, Cooking time: 0 minutes, Servings: 2

Ingredients

- Medium avocado, pitted and scooped – ½
- Spinach, fresh – ½ cup
- Erythritol sweetener – 2 tbsp
- Vanilla powder – ½ tsp
- MCT oil – 1 tbsp
- Coconut milk, unsweetened – ½ cup
- Ice cubes – ½ cup
- Water – ½ cup

Instructions

1. Place all the ingredients for smoothie in a blender and pulse for 1 to 2 minutes or until smooth.
2. Divide smoothie evenly between two glasses and serve.

Nutritional facts

Calories: 256; Fat: 26.4g; Saturated fat: 18g; Net Carbohydrate: 13.4g; Protein: 2.4g; Fiber: 4.2g;

Green Breakfast Smoothie

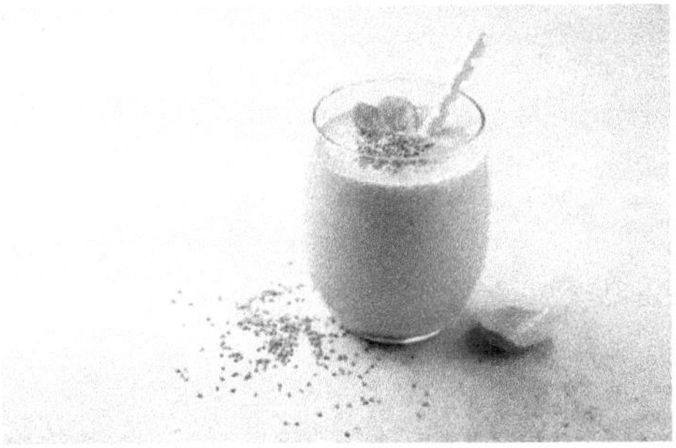

Prep time: 5 minutes, Cooking time: 0 minutes, Servings: 2

Ingredients

- Spinach – 2 oz
- Almond milk, unsweetened – 3 cups
- Medium avocado, pitted and scooped – 3.5 oz
- Cucumber – 3.5 oz
- Celery – 3.5 oz
- Chia seeds – 1 tsp
- Matcha powder – 2 tsp
- Protein powder – 2 scoop
- Liquid stevia – 20 drops
- Coconut oil – 2 tbsps

Instructions

1. Place spinach and almond milk in a blender and pulse for 1 minute or until spinach break down.
2. Then add remaining ingredients into the blender and pulse for 1 to 2 minutes or until smooth.
3. Divide smoothie evenly between two glasses and serve.

Nutritional facts

Calories: 375; Fat: 25g; Saturated fat: 15g; Net Carbohydrate: 4g; Protein: 30g; Fiber: 3g;

Cinnamon Almond Butter Shake

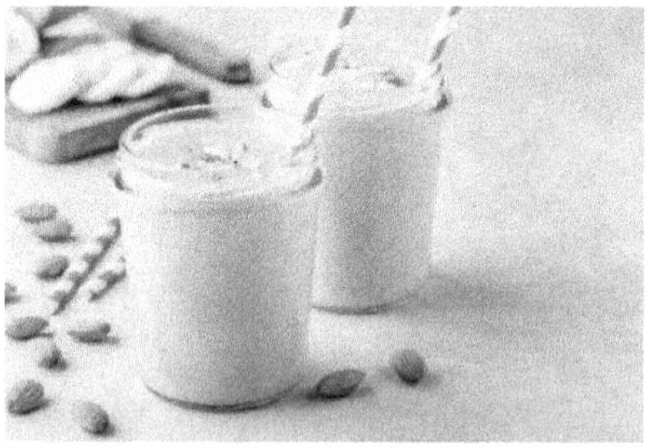

Prep time: 5 minutes, Cooking time: 0 minutes, Servings: 2

Ingredients

- Golden flax meal – 4 tbsp
- Cinnamon – 1 tsp
- Collagen peptides – 2 scoops
- Salt – ¼ tsp
- Liquid stevia – 30 drops
- Almond extract – ¼ tsp
- Almond butter – 4 tbsp
- Almond milk, unsweetened – 3 cups
- Ice cubes – 1 cup

Instructions

1. Place all the ingredients in a blender and pulse for 1 to 2 minutes or until smooth.
2. Divide shake evenly between two glasses and serve.

Nutritional facts

Calories: 326; Fat: 27g; Saturated fat: 19g; Net Carbohydrate: 6g; Protein: 19g; Fiber: 5g;

Beetroot Shake

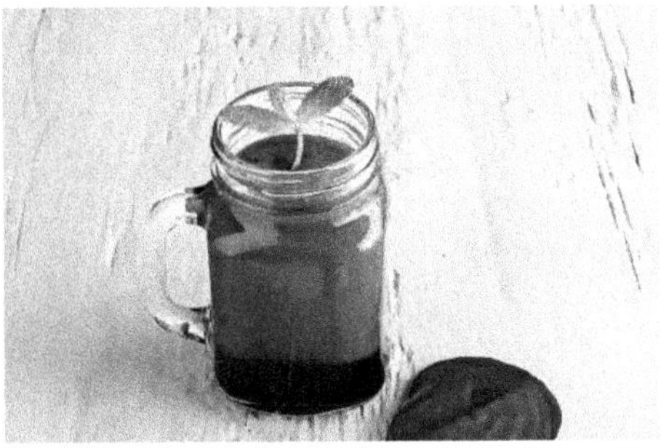

Prep time: 5 minutes, Cooking time: 0 minutes, Servings: 2

Ingredients

- Cinnamon – ½ tsp
- Whey protein – 2 scoops
- Beetroot powder – 2 tsp
- Vanilla extract, unsweetened – 2 tsp
- MCT oil – 2 tbsp
- Coconut milk, unsweetened – 2 cups

Instructions

1. Place all the ingredients in a blender and pulse for 1 minute or until smooth.
2. Divide shake evenly between two glasses and serve.

Nutritional facts

Calories: 300; Fat: 12g; Saturated fat: 18g; Net Carbohydrate: 3g; Protein: 25g; Fiber: 3g;

Chocolate Peanut Butter Smoothie

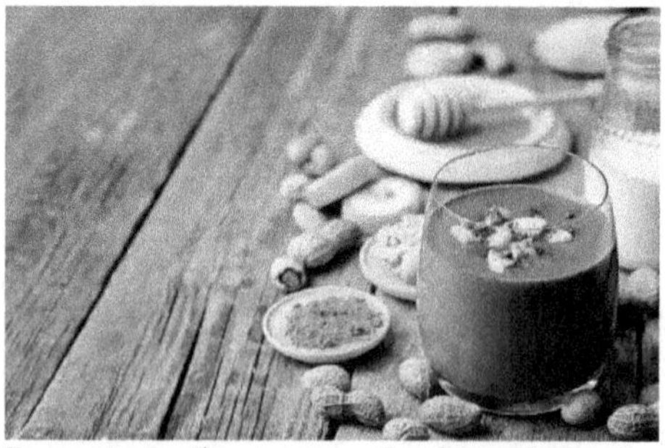

Prep time: 5 minutes, Cooking time: 0 minutes, Servings: 2

Ingredients

- Peanut butter – 3 tbsp
- Erythritol sweetener – 4 tbsp
- Cocoa powder – 2 tbsp
- Heavy cream – ¾ cup
- Almond milk, unsweetened – 1 cup

Instructions

1. Place all the ingredients in a blender and pulse for 1 minute or until smooth.
2. Divide shake evenly between two glasses and serve.

Nutritional facts

Calories: 435; Fat: 41g; Saturated fat: 28g; Net Carbohydrate: 4g; Protein: 9g; Fiber: 6g;

Chapter 3 Lunch

Garlic Chicken

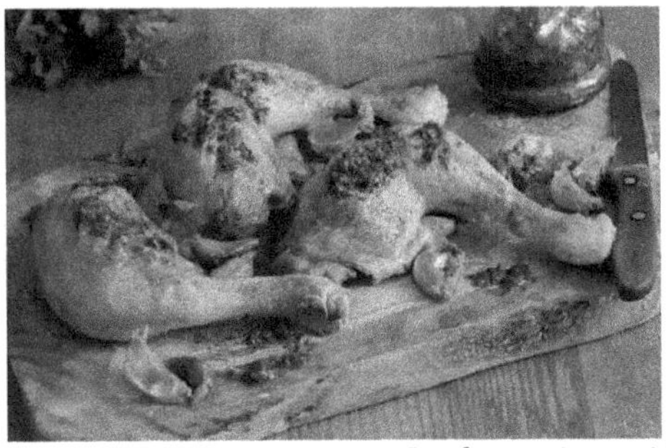

Prep time: 10 minutes, Cooking time: 40 minutes, Servings: 2

Ingredients

- Chicken thighs - 1 pound
- Salt - 1 ½ tsp
- Ground black pepper - 1 tsp
- Minced garlic - 3½ tsp
- Lemon, the juice - ½
- Chopped fresh parsley - ¼ cup
- Butter - 2 tbsp
- Olive oil - 1 tbsp

Instructions

1. Set oven to 450 ° F and let preheat.
2. Meanwhile, take a baking pan, grease it with butter, then add chicken and season with salt and black pepper.
3. Drizzle chicken with lemon juice and oil and sprinkle with garlic and parsley.
4. Place baking pan into the oven and bake for 30 to 40 minutes or until chicken is no longer pink and cooked.

Nutritional facts

Calories: 543; Fat: 39g; Saturated fat: 27g; Net Carbohydrate: 3g; Protein: 42g; Fiber: 1g;

Buffalo drumsticks

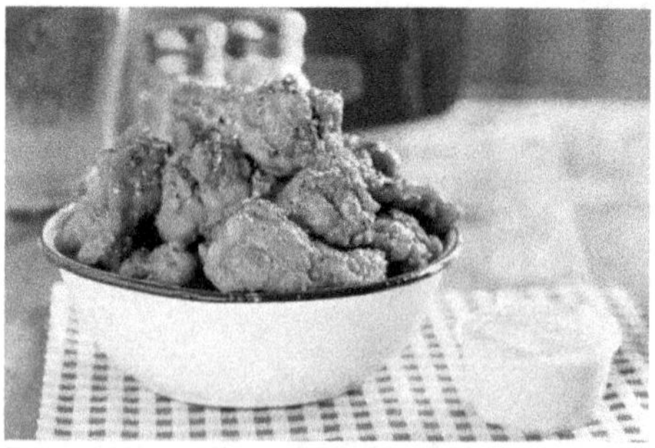

Prep time: 15 minutes, Cooking time: 40 minutes, Servings: 2

Ingredients

For Aioli:

- Mayonnaise - 51/3 tbsp
- Smoked paprika - ½ tbsp
- Minced garlic - ½ tsp

For Drumsticks:

- Chicken drumsticks - 1 pound
- Salt - ½ tsp
- Paprika powder - ½ tsp
- Tabasco sauce - ½ tbsp
- Tomato paste - ½ tbsp
- White wine vinegar - 1 tbsp
- Olive oil - 1 tbsp

Instructions

1. Set oven to 450 ° F and let preheat.
2. Meanwhile, place drumsticks in a large plastic bag, then whisk together remaining ingredients for drumsticks until smooth and pour over drumsticks.
3. Seal the plastic bag, then turn it upside down until drumsticks are evenly coated with the mixture and then let marinate for 10 minutes.
4. Then take a large baking dish, grease with oil and place marinated chicken drumsticks on it.
5. Place baking dish into the oven and bake the chicken for 30 to 40 minutes or until chicken is no longer pink and done.
6. In the meantime, prepared aioli and for this, whisk together all the ingredients for aioli in a bowl until combined.
7. Serve chicken drumsticks with prepared aioli.

Nutritional facts

Calories: 692; Fat: 56g; Saturated fat: 41g; Net Carbohydrate: 2g; Protein: 42g; Fiber: 1g;

Chicken Philly Cheesesteak Casserole

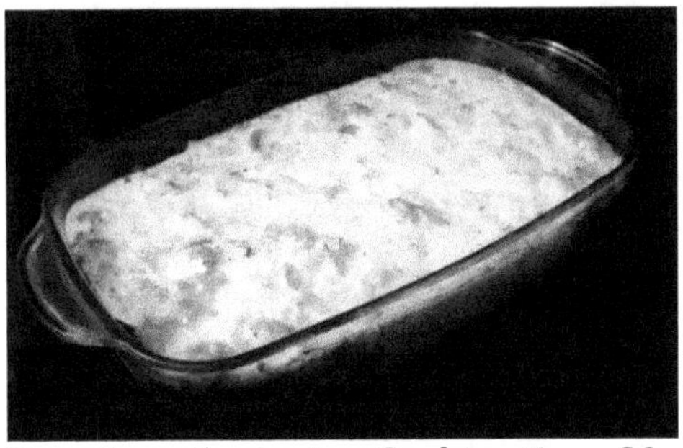

Prep time: 5 minutes, Cooking time: 30 minutes, Servings: 2

Ingredients

- Chicken breasts, 1-inch cubed - 2/3 pound
- Green bell peppers, sliced - 1/3 cup
- Mushrooms, sliced - 2 2/3 oz
- Medium white onions, sliced - 1/3 cup
- Minced garlic - ½ teaspoon
- Salt - 1/6 tsp
- Ground black pepper - 1/6 tsp
- Italian seasoning, divided - 2/3 tsp
- Worcestershire sauce - 2/3 tbsp
- Butter - 1/3 tbsp
- Grated cheddar cheese - 2/3 cup
- Cream cheese, softened - 2 2/3 oz
- Provolone cheese slices - 4 oz
- Mayonnaise - 1/6 cup

Instructions

1. Set oven to 375 ^{o} F and let preheat.
2. Meanwhile, take a large skillet pan, place it over medium heat, add butter and when it melts, add chicken and cook for 7 to 10 minutes until chicken golden brown.
3. Meanwhile, place cream cheese in a bowl, add ¼ teaspoon garlic, 1/3 teaspoon Italian seasoning, Worcestershire sauce, mayonnaise and cheese and whisk until combined, set aside until required.
4. Add remaining ingredients into the cooked chicken, except for provolone cheese slices, and cook for 3 minutes or until vegetables are tender-crisp.
5. Spoon the chicken mixture into cream cheese mixture and stir until combined.
6. Take a 9 by 13-inch baking dish, add chicken mixture, spread evenly and then top with cheese slices.
7. Place baking dish into the oven and bake for 15 to 20 minutes or until the top is nicely golden brown and the mixture is bubbly.
8. Serve straight away.

Nutritional facts

Calories: 489; Fat: 40g; Saturated fat: 28g; Net Carbohydrate: 5g; Protein: 26g; Fiber: 1g;

Butter Chicken

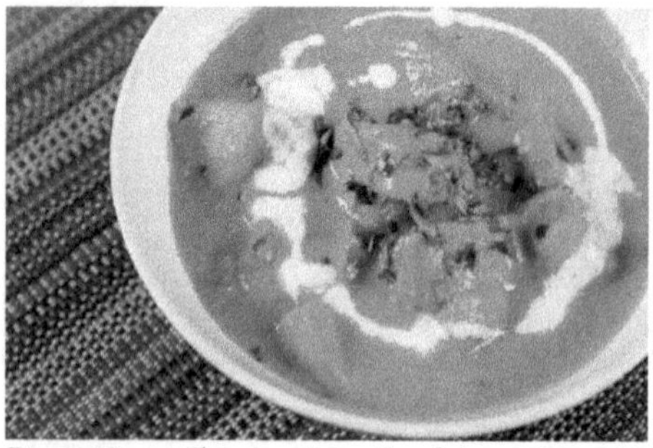

Prep time: 5 minutes, Cooking time: 18 minutes, Servings: 2

Ingredients

- Chicken breast, 1-inch cubed – ½ pound
- Medium white onion, peeled and sliced – 1/8
- Minced garlic – ¼ tsp
- Ginger powder – ½ tsp
- Salt – ½ tsp
- Red chili powder – ½ tsp
- Turmeric powder – ¾ tsp
- Ground cinnamon – ¼ tsp
- Tomato paste – ¾ tbsp
- Butter – 1 tbsp
- Heavy whipping cream – ½ cup

Instructions

1. Place chicken in a bowl, add ginger, salt, red chili powder, turmeric, and cinnamon and toss until well coated.
2. Place a skillet over medium heat, add butter and when it melts, add onion and garlic and cook for 2 to 3 minutes or until onions are translucent.
3. Increase heat to medium-high level, add the seasoned chicken and cook for 5 minutes or until chicken is no longer pink and nicely golden brown.
4. Switch heat to a medium low level, then add tomato paste and cream, stir until mixed, and simmer chicken for 5 to 7 minutes or until chicken is cooked fully.
5. Cook chicken curry more for 1 to 2 minutes or until curry is slightly thick.
6. Serve curry with cooked cauliflower rice.

Nutritional facts

Calories: 385; Fat: 26.7g; Saturated fat: 18.2g; Net Carbohydrate: 4.3g; Protein: 26.5g; Fiber: 1.2g;

Turkey Soup

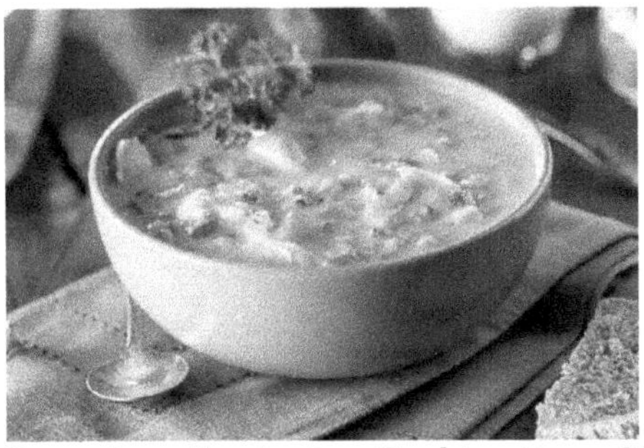

Prep time: 5 minutes, Cooking time: 20 minutes, Servings: 2

Ingredients

- Frozen riced cauliflower - 6 oz
- Leftover chopped turkey - ½ pound
- Celery stalks, diced small - 1 medium
- White mushrooms, chopped - ½ cup
- Red onion, diced small - ¼ cup
- Italian seasoning - ½ tbsp
- Onion powder - ¼ tsp
- Garlic powder - ¼ tsp
- Sea salt - ½ teaspoon
- Ground black pepper - ¼ teaspoon
- Crushed red pepper flakes - ¼ tsp
- Chopped parsley - 1 ½ tbsp
- Olive oil - 1 tbsp
- Chicken broth - 3 cups
- Heavy cream - ¼ cup
- Shredded Italian blend cheese - 1 cup

Instructions

1. Place a large skillet pan over medium-high heat, add oil and when hot, add onion and celery and cook for 5 minutes or until softened.
2. Add remaining ingredients, except for cauliflower rice, broth, cream, and cheese, stir well and cook for 7 minutes.
3. Pour in broth, simmer the soup for 3 minutes or until heated, then whisk together cream and 1 tablespoon cooking liquid, add it into the pan and stir well.
4. Simmer the soup for 2 minutes, then add cauliflower rice and ¾ cup cheese, stir until combined and cook for another 2 minutes or until cauliflower is well heated.
5. Remove pan from heat, ladle soup into bowl and top with remaining cheese.
6. Serve straight away.

Nutritional facts

Calories: 409; Fat: 30.4g; Saturated fat: 14g; Net Carbohydrate: 4.1g; Protein: 26.6g; Fiber: 3g;

Grilled Fish with Zucchini and Pesto

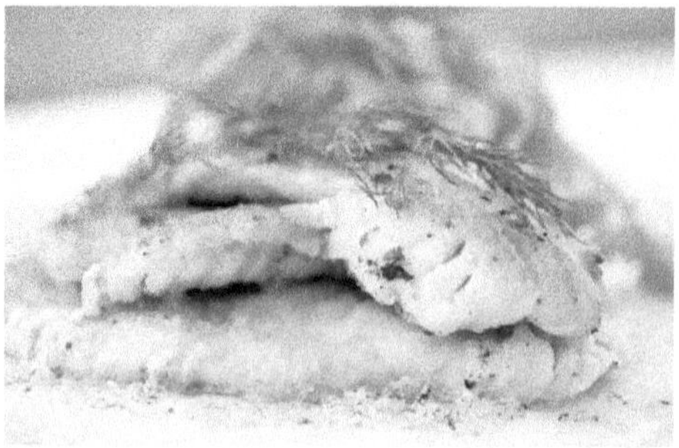

Prep time: 10 minutes, Cooking time: 8 minutes, Servings: 2

Ingredients

For Fish and Zucchini:

- Whitefish – ¾ pound
- Medium size zucchini, thinly sliced – 1
- Salt – 1 tsp
- Ground black pepper – ½ tsp
- Lemon juice – ½ tbsp
- Olive oil – 1 tbsp

For Kale Pesto:

- Kale leaves – 1½ oz
- Walnuts – 1 oz
- Minced garlic – ¼ tsp
- Salt – ¼ tsp
- Ground black pepper – 1/8 tsp
- Lemon juice – 1½ tbsp
- Olive oil – 2/5 cup

Instructions

1. Prepare kale pesto and for this, place all the ingredients for the kale pesto in a food processor and pulse for 1 to 2 minutes or until smooth.
2. Tip pesto in a bowl and set aside until required.
3. Place zucchini slices in a bowl, season with ½ teaspoon salt and ¼ teaspoon black pepper, drizzle with lemon juice and olive oil and toss until evenly coated, set aside until required.
4. Season fish with remaining salt and black pepper and let sit for 5 minutes.
5. Meanwhile, place a frying pan over medium heat, grease with oil and let preheat.
6. Pat dry fish with paper towels, brush with oil and add to the frying pan to cook for 3 to 5 minutes per side.
7. When done, serve fish with zucchini and pesto.

Nutritional facts

Calories: 778; Fat: 67g; Saturated fat: 3g; Net Carbohydrate: 7g; Protein: 38g; Fiber: 3g;

Salmon Meatballs

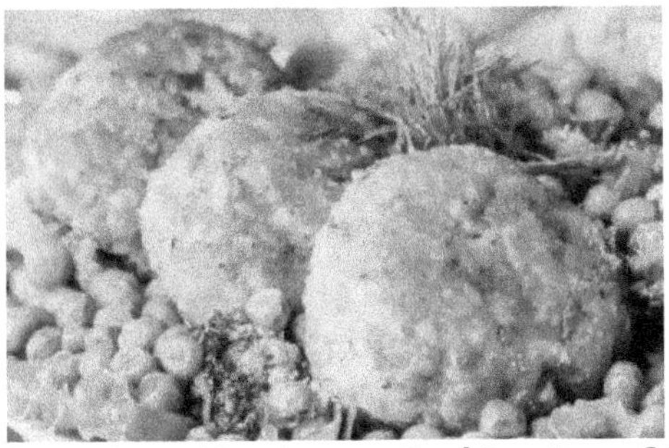

Prep time: 10 minutes, Cooking time: 20 minutes, Servings: 2

Ingredients

The Meatballs:

- Salmon skinless and cut into 1-inch pieces – 1 pound
- Medium white onion, grated – ½
- Minced cilantro – 3 tbsp
- Minced garlic – 1 tsp
- Salt – ¾ tsp
- Ground pepper – ½ tsp
- Paprika – ½ tsp
- Ground oregano – ½ tsp
- Egg white – 1
- Panko breadcrumbs – ¼ cup and 2 tbsp

The Sauce:

- Medium avocado, pitted and scooped – 1
- Minced garlic – ½ tsp
- Minced cilantro – 2 tbsp
- Salt – ¼ tsp
- Ground black pepper – ¼ tsp
- Chipotle chili powder – ½ tsp
- Lime, juiced – ½
- Greek yogurt – 3 tbsp
- Water – 5 tbsp

Instructions

1. Set oven to 350 ^{o} F and let preheat.
2. Meanwhile, prepare meatballs and for this, place salmon in a food processor and pulse for 1 to 2 minutes or until finely chopped.
3. Tip the chopped salmon into a large bowl, add remaining ingredients for meatballs and stir until combined.
4. Shape mixture into four meatballs and then place on a baking sheet greased with oil.
5. Place the baking sheet into the oven and bake for 18 minutes or until nicely golden brown and cooked.
6. In the meantime, prepare the sauce and for this, place all the ingredients for the sauce in a blender and pulse for 1 to 2 minutes or until smooth.
7. Tip the avocado sauce in a bowl and serve.

Nutritional facts

Calories: 295; Fat: 12.7g; Saturated fat: 2.4g; Net Carbohydrate: 7g; Protein: 35g; Fiber: 3g;

Fried Salmon with Green Beans

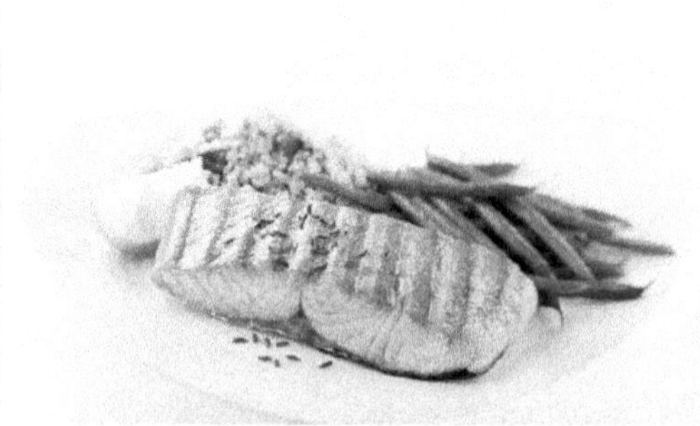

Prep time: 5 minutes, Cooking time: 8 minutes, Servings: 2

Ingredients

- Green beans, trimmed – 9 oz
- Salmon, cut into pieces – 9 oz
- Salt – ½ tsp
- Ground black pepper – ½ tsp
- Coconut oil – 3½ oz

Instructions

1. Place a frying pan over medium heat, add oil and when hot, add beans and cook for 4 minutes.
2. Season beans with salt and black pepper, move them to one side and place salmon on the empty side of the pan.
3. Cook salmon for 3 to 4 minutes per side until nicely golden brown on all side, stirring beans frequently.
4. When done, slide salmon and beans to a plate, season salmon with salt and black pepper and serve.

Nutritional facts

Calories: 657; Fat: 58g; Saturated fat: 41g; Net Carbohydrate: 5g; Protein: 28g; Fiber: 3g;

Garlic Butter Salmon

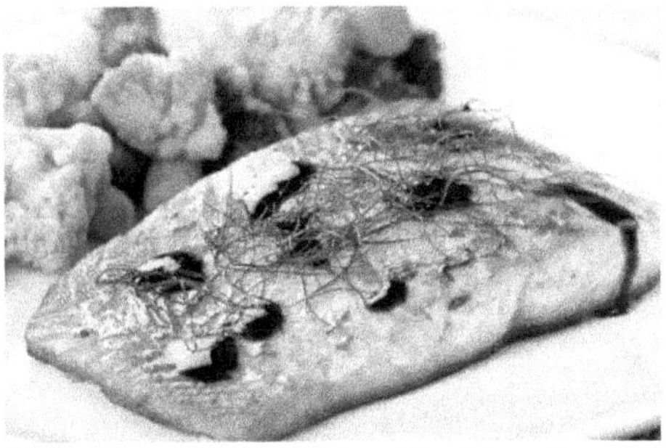

Prep time: 10 minutes, Cooking time: 22 minutes, Servings: 2

Ingredients

- Salmon filet, cut into 4 pieces – ¾ pound
- Cauliflower florets – ½ pound
- Minced garlic – 1 tsp
- Salt – 1 tsp
- Ground black pepper – ½ tsp
- Chopped parsley – 1 tbsp
- Lemon zest – ½ tsp
- Butter, soften – 1 tbsp
- Butter, melted – 1 tbsp
- Lemon wedges for serving

Instructions

1. Set oven to 400 ° F, then grease a rimmed baking sheet with butter, place it into the oven and let preheat.
2. Place melted butter in a small bowl, add garlic, lemon zest and parsley and whisk until combined.
3. Spread cauliflower florets on a heated baking sheet, sprinkle with ½ teaspoon salt and ¼ teaspoon black pepper and toss until coated.
4. Return baking sheet into the oven and bake for 10 minutes.
5. Then push florets to one side of the baking sheet, place salmon fillet to the other side of the sheet, sprinkle salmon with remaining salt and black pepper on both side and then drizzle with the butter garlic mixture.
6. Return baking sheet into the oven and continue baking for 10 to 12 minutes or until fish is cooked through.
7. Serve salmon and cauliflower florets with lemon wedges.

Nutritional facts

Calories: 450; Fat: 24g; Saturated fat: 16g; Net Carbohydrate: 6.3g; Protein: 40g; Fiber: 2.4g;

Sesame Salmon with Thai Curry Cabbage

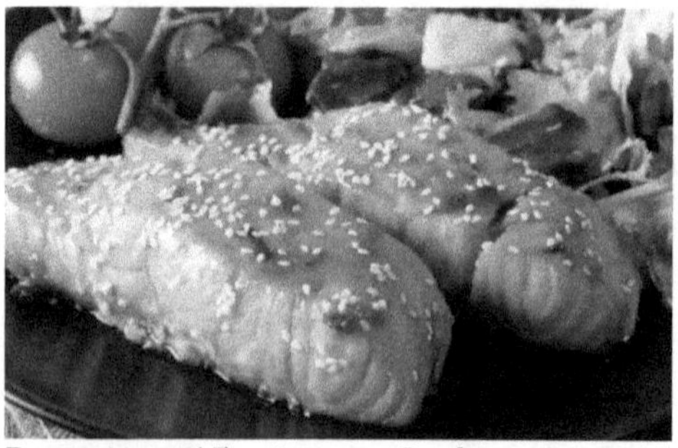

Prep time: 15 minutes, Cooking time: 15 minutes, Servings: 2

Ingredients

Thai curry cabbage

- Shredded green cabbage - 15 oz
- Salt - ½ tsp
- Ground black pepper - ¼ tsp
- Red curry paste - ½ tbsp
- Sesame oil - ½ tbsp
- Coconut oil - 1 tbsp

Lime mayo

- Lime, juiced and zested - ¼
- Mayonnaise - ½ cup
- Salt - 1/8 tsp

Salmon

- Salmon - 12 oz
- Salt - ¾ tsp
- Ground black pepper - ½ tsp
- Sesame seeds - 1 tbsp
- Butter - 1½ oz
- Lime, for serving - ½

Instructions

1. Prepare lime mayonnaise and for this, place all its ingredients in a bowl and whisk until combined, refrigerate sauce until required.
2. Prepare curry cabbage and for this, place a frying pan over high heat, add coconut oil and when hot, add cabbage and stir in curry paste.
3. Cook cabbage for 3 to 5 minutes or until sauté, then season with salt and black pepper, drizzle with sesame oil and remove the pan from heat.
4. Transfer cabbage to a bowl, cover it and set aside until required, keep cabbage warm.
5. Prepare salmon and for this, cut salmon into pieces, season with salt and black pepper until evenly coated and then press into sesame seeds.
6. Return frying pan over medium-high heat, add butter and when it melts, add salmon pieces.
7. Baste salmon with melted butter and cook for 3 minutes per side or until cooked.
8. Serve salmon with curry cabbage and lime mayonnaise.

Nutritional facts

Calories: 544; Fat: 48g; Saturated fat: 27g; Net Carbohydrate: 4.5g; Protein: 20g; Fiber: 3.5g;

BBQ Ribs

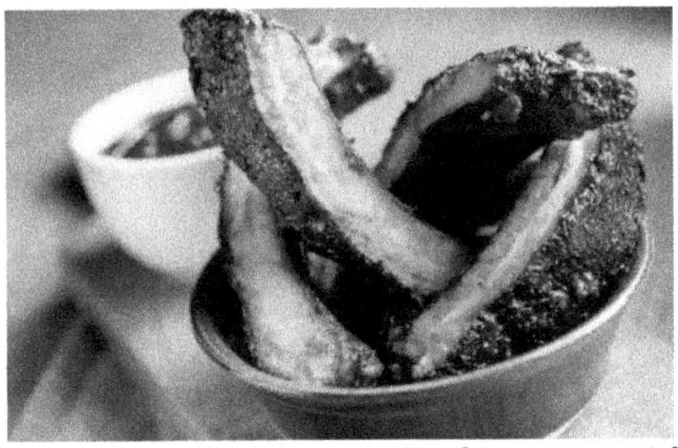

Prep time: 10 minutes, Cooking time: 1 hour and 35 minutes, Servings: 2

Ingredients

For Rubs:

- Onion powder - 1/3 tsp
- Garlic powder - 1/3 tsp
- Salt - 1/3 tbsp
- Ground black pepper - 1/3 tsp
- Red chili powder - 1/3 tbsp
- Paprika - 1/3 tbsp
- Cayenne pepper - 1/8 tsp
- Dried oregano - 1/3 tsp

Ribs:

- Pork spare ribs - 1/3 rack
- BBQ sauce, unsweetened - 3 tbsp
- Water - 1/3 cup

Instructions

1. Set oven to 425 ^{o} F and let preheat.
2. Meanwhile, stir all the ingredients for the rub in a bowl until mixed and then sprinkle and rub it generously on all sides of pork ribs until evenly coated.
3. Place seasoned ribs on a roasting pan, pour water in it and then cover the pan with aluminum foil.
4. Place roasting pan into the oven and bake for 1 hour and 30 minutes or until ribs are tender.
5. Then transfer ribs onto a baking sheet, brush them with BBQ sauce and cook ribs under the broiler for 3 minutes or more until nicely browned.
6. Serve straight away.

Nutritional facts

Calories: 455; Fat: 31g; Saturated fat: 19g; Net Carbohydrate: 1.3g; Protein: 33.2g; Fiber: 0.5g;

Stuffed Zucchini Boats

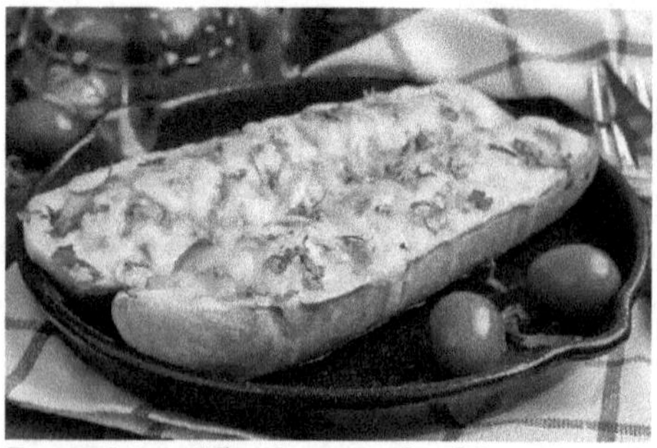

Prep time: 15 minutes, Cooking time: 30 minutes, Servings: 2

Ingredients

- Ground beef - ½ pound
- Medium zucchini - 1
- Salt, divided - ¾ tsp
- Ground black pepper - ¼ tsp
- Tex-Mex seasoning - 1 tbsp
- Chopped cilantro - 2 tbsp
- Olive oil, divided - 1 tbsp
- Grated mozzarella cheese - 2/3 cup

Instructions

1. Set oven to 400 ° F and let preheat.
2. Meanwhile, cut zucchini in half, remove its seeds, then sprinkle with ½ teaspoon salt and let zucchini sit for 10 minutes.
3. In the meantime, place a skillet pan over medium heat, add 1 tablespoon oil and when hot, add ground beef to cook for 5 minutes or more until nicely browned.
4. Season beef with salt and Tex-Mex seasoning and cook for 3 minutes or until all the cooking liquid is evaporated.
5. Pat dry zucchini with paper towels, then add cilantro and 1/3 cup of cheese in beef mixture, stir well and then stuff the beef mixture into zucchini halves.
6. Sprinkle remaining cheese on top of stuffed zucchini and place on a baking sheet greased with oil.
7. Place the baking sheet into the oven and bake zucchini for 20 minutes or until the top is nicely browned.
8. Serve straight away.

Nutritional facts

Calories: 300; Fat: 25g; Saturated fat: 17g; Net Carbohydrate: 3g; Protein: 16g; Fiber: 1.5g;

Sesame Salmon with Bok Choy

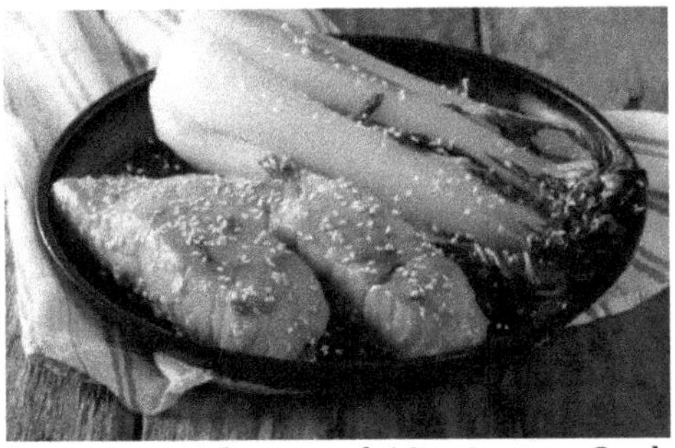

Prep time: 1 hour and 10 minutes, Cooking time: 20 minutes, Servings: 2

Ingredients

- Salmon fillet – 2, each about 4 ounce
- Portobello mushroom cap, ½-inch diced – 1
- Small green onion – 1
- Baby bok choy, ends trimmed – 2
- Sesame seeds, toasted – ½ tbsp

Marinade

- Grated ginger – ½ tsp
- Salt – ¼ tsp
- Ground black pepper – ¼ tsp
- Coconut aminos – ½ tbsp
- Lemon juice – ¼ tsp
- Olive oil – ½ tbsp
- Sesame oil – ½ tsp

Instructions

1. Place all the ingredients for the marinade in a bowl and whisk until combined.
2. Place salmon fillet in a plastic bag, pour in half of the marinade, then seal the bag and turn it upside and down to coat salmon with the marinade and marinate in the refrigerator for 1 hour.
3. When ready to cook, set the oven to 400 ° F and let preheat.
4. Cut bok choy in half, then place on a baking sheet, add mushrooms, drizzle with remaining marinade and toss until mixed.
5. Add marinated salmon to the baking sheet and bake for 20 minutes or until salmon is cooked through.
6. When done, evenly divide salmon, mushrooms and bok choy between plates, sprinkle with sesame seeds and serve.

Nutritional facts

Calories: 167; Fat: 10g; Saturated fat: 3g; Net Carbohydrate: 1.1g; Protein: 17g; Fiber: 1.2g;

Tuna Stuffed Tomatoes

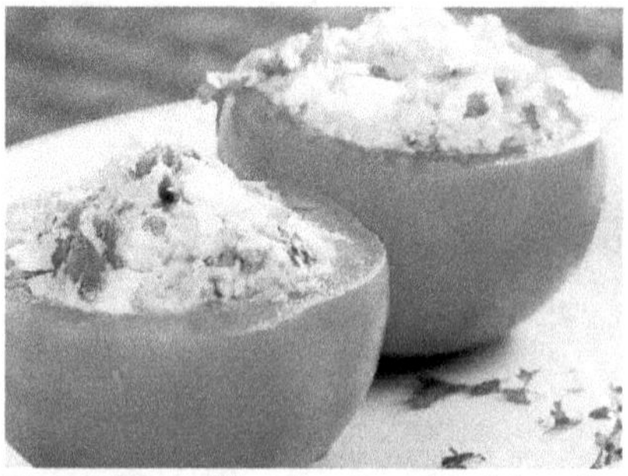

Prep time: 10 minutes, Cooking time: 0 minutes, Servings: 2

Ingredients

- Cooked tuna, flaked – 12 ounces
- Celery ribs, chopped – 2
- Celery salt – ½ teaspoon
- Ground black pepper – ¼ teaspoon
- Dill weed – ½ teaspoon
- Mayonnaise – ½ cup

Instructions

1. Cut the top of the tomato, about a ¼ inch and then remove the seeds from inside.
2. Place remaining ingredients, except for sour cream, in a bowl, stir until well mixed and then stuff the mixture into tomatoes.
3. Serve immediately.

Nutritional facts

Calories: 241; Fat: 11g; Saturated fat: 2g; Net Carbohydrate: 6g; Protein: 24g; Fiber: 5g;

Pork Carnitas

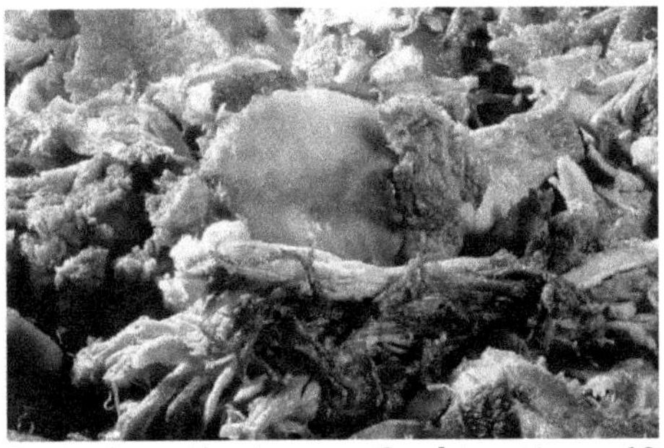

Prep time: 5 minutes, Cooking time: 60 minutes, Servings: 2

Ingredients

- Pork shoulder, fat trimmed – 1 pound
- Orange, halved – ½
- Jalapeño, deseeded and diced – 1 small
- Medium white onion, peeled and diced – ½
- Minced garlic – ¾ tsp
- Salt – 1 tsp
- Ground black pepper – ¼ tsp
- Paprika – ½ tsp
- Ground cumin – ¼ tsp
- Dried parsley – ½ tsp
- Limes, juiced – 1
- Olive oil – 1 tbsp
- Water – ½ cup

Instructions

1. Cut pork into large pieces and season with salt and black pepper.
2. Plugin the instant pot, grease the inner pot with oil, press the 'sauté' button and when oil is hot, add seasoned pork and cook for 5 minutes per side or until seared.
3. Press the cancel button, add remaining ingredients and toss until mixed.
4. Shut instant pot with lid, press 'meat' button and cook for 30 minutes at high pressure.
5. When the instant pot beep, do natural pressure release, then open the instant pot and shred pork with two forks.
6. Transfer shredded pork to a rimmed baking sheet, spread evenly, then drizzle with some of the cooking liquid from the inner pot and broil for 5 to 7 minutes or until edges begin to crispy.
7. Serve straight away.

Nutritional facts

Calories: 272; Fat: 15g; Saturated fat: 4g; Net Carbohydrate: 2g; Protein: 30g; Fiber: 0g;

Chapter 4 Snacks and sides

Caesar salad

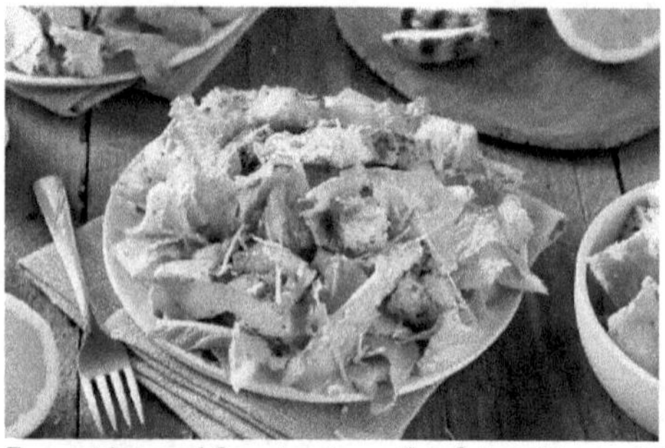

Prep time: 10 minutes, Cooking time: 20 minutes, Servings: 2

Ingredients

For Dressing

- Mayonnaise – ½ cup
- Dijon mustard – 1 tbsp
- Lemon, zest, and juice – ½
- Grated parmesan cheese – 2 tbsp
- Chopped anchovies – 2 tbsp
- Salt – ¼ tsp
- Ground black pepper – ¼ tsp

For Salad

- Chicken breasts – ¾ pound
- Bacon, chopped – 3 oz
- Romaine lettuce, chopped – 7 oz
- Salt – 1 tsp
- Ground black pepper – ½ tsp
- Olive oil – 1 tbsp
- Grated parmesan cheese – 1 oz

Instructions

1. Set oven to 350 ° F and let preheat.
2. Meanwhile, prepare the dressing and for this, place all the ingredients for dressing in a bowl, whisk using an immersion blender until smooth and set aside.
3. Prepare salad and for this, season chicken with salt and black pepper and place in a greased baking dish.
4. Drizzle oil on the chicken, then place the baking dish into the oven and bake for 20 minutes or until chicken is no longer pink and cooked through, slice when done.
5. In the meantime, place a frying pan over medium heat, add bacon and cook for 3 minutes per side until crispy, set aside until required.
6. To assemble the salad, divide chopped cabbage evenly between two plates, top with chicken slices and bacon pieces and drizzle with prepared dressing.
7. Garnish salad with parmesan cheese and serve.

Nutritional facts

Calories: 1027; Fat: 88g; Saturated fat: 58g; Net Carbohydrate: 4g; Protein: 52g; Fiber: 3g;

Lemon Lamb Skewers

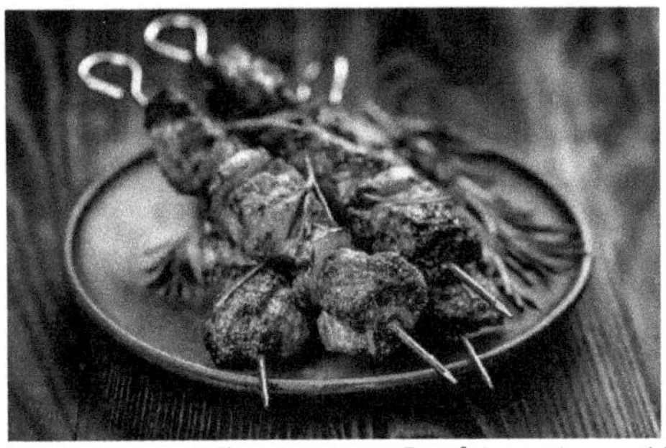

Prep time: 15 minutes, Cooking time: 15 minutes, Servings: 2

Ingredients

- Lamb roasts, boneless - ¾ pound
- Salt - 1 tsp
- Ground black pepper - ½ tsp
- Dried oregano - ½ tbsp
- Dried rosemary - ½ tbsp
- Dried parsley - ½ tbsp
- Lemon, zested - ½
- Lemon juice - ½ tbsp
- Olive oil - 1 tbsp

For Aioli

- Minced garlic - ½ tsp
- Salt - ¼ tsp
- Ground black pepper - ¼ tsp
- Lemon juice - ½ tbsp
- Mayonnaise - 1/3 cup

Instructions

1. Cut lamb roast into small pieces and place in a bowl, add remaining ingredients, toss well until evenly coated and marinate for 10 minutes.
2. Meanwhile, prepare aioli and for this, whisk together all the ingredients for aioli until combined, set aside until required.
3. Prepare grill, then brush the grilling rack with oil and preheat at high heat setting.
4. Thread marinated lamb pieces in soaked wooden skewers, place them on grilling rack and grill for 15 minutes or until cooked.
5. Serve lamb skewers with prepared aioli.

Nutritional facts

Calories: 913; Fat: 81g; Saturated fat: 57g; Net Carbohydrate: 4g; Protein: 10g; Fiber: 2g;

Shrimp Salad

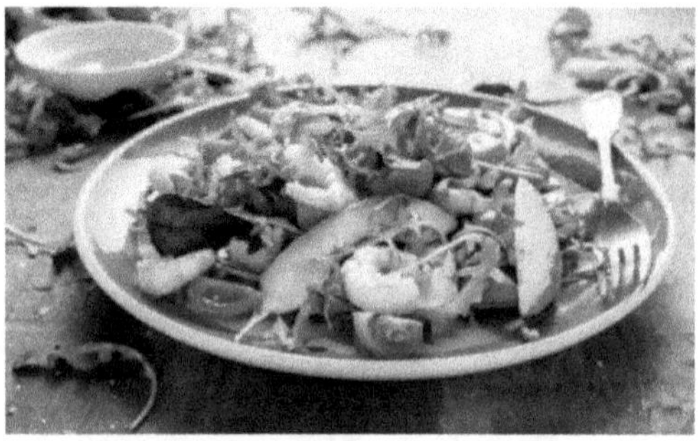

Prep time: 10 minutes, Cooking time: 5 minutes, Servings: 2

Ingredients

- Shrimp, peeled and deveined – 10 oz
- Medium avocados, pitted and scooped – 2
- Cucumber – 5 oz
- Baby spinach – 2 oz
- Salt, divided – 1 tsp
- Lime, juiced – ½
- Minced garlic – 1 tsp
- Red chili powder – 2 tsp
- Olive oil – 3 tbsp

Ginger dressing

- Avocado oil – ¼ cup
- Grated ginger – 1 tbsp
- Lime, juice – ½
- Soy sauce – ½ tbsp
- Minced garlic – ¼ tsp
- Salt – ¼ tsp
- Ground black pepper – ¼ tsp

Instructions

1. Slice scooped avocado flesh and add it into a bowl along with cucumber and spinach, season with ½ salt, drizzle with lime juice, then toss until combined and set aside until required.
2. Place a skillet pan over medium heat, add oil and when hot, add garlic and red chili powder and fry for 1 minute or until fragrant.
3. Add shrimps into the skillet pan and cook for 3 to 4 minutes or until opaque.
4. Remove pan from the heat, season shrimps with remaining salt and black pepper and add to the salad bowl.
5. Prepare the dressing and for this, place all the ingredients for the ginger dressing in a bowl and whisk with an immersion blender until combined.
6. Drizzle the dressing over shrimps and serve.

Nutritional facts

Calories: 871; Fat: 79g; Saturated fat: 62g; Net Carbohydrate: 9g; Protein: 26g; Fiber: 16g;

Zucchini Salmon Fritters

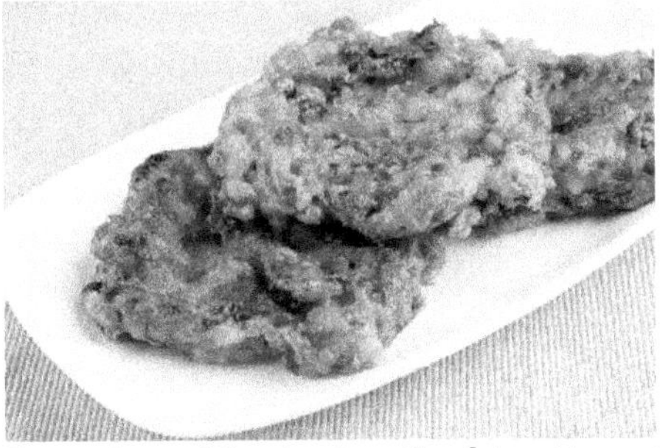

Prep time: 10 minutes, Cooking time: 6 minutes, Servings: 2

Ingredients

For Zucchini Salmon Fritters

- Cooked salmon, flaked - 7½ oz
- Medium zucchini, grated - ½
- White onions, chopped - 1 tbsp
- Salt - ½ tsp
- Ground black pepper - ¼ tsp
- Ground Psyllium husk powder - ½ tbsp
- Egg - ½
- Butter - 2¼ oz

For Tartar Sauce

- Scallions, minced - ½ tbsp
- Horseradish - 1 tsp
- Dill pickle, minced - ½
- Salt - ¼ tsp
- Ground black pepper - ¼ tsp
- Apple cider vinegar - 1 tsp
- Mayonnaise - ½ tbsp
- Greek yogurt - ½ tbsp
- Heavy whipping cream - ¼ tbsp

Instructions

1. Prepare fritters and for this, place salmon in a bowl, add zucchini and onion, season with salt and black pepper, sprinkle with Psyllium husk and add the egg.
2. Stir all the ingredients in a bowl until well combined and then evenly shape in small bowls, set aside until required.
3. Prepare tartar sauce and for this, place all the ingredients for tartar sauce in a bowl, stir until well mixed and set aside until required.
4. Place a frying pan over medium heat, add butter and when it melts, add fritters, then flatten them slightly to make round fritters and cook for 3 minutes per side or more until nicely golden brown on all sides.
5. Serve fritters with prepared tartar sauce.

Nutritional facts

Calories: 523; Fat: 45g; Saturated fat: 31g; Net Carbohydrate: 3g; Protein: 25g; Fiber: 3g;

Lamb Sliders

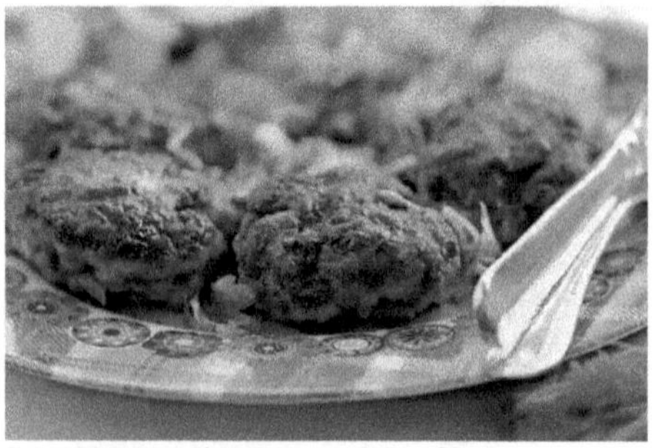

Prep time: 5 minutes, Cooking time: 8 minutes, Servings: 2

Ingredients

- Ground lamb – ½ pound
- Medium white onion, peeled and diced – 1/8
- Minced garlic – ½ tsp
- Sea salt – ¼ tsp
- Ground black pepper – ¼ tsp
- Dried oregano – 1 tsp
- Lemon, zested – ½
- Olive oil – 2 tbsp

Instructions

1. Place all the ingredients in a bowl, except for oil, stir until well mixed and then shape mixture into four patties.
2. Place a skillet pan over medium heat, add oil and when hot, add patties and cook for 3 to 4 minutes per side or until nicely golden brown and cooked.
3. Serve straight away.

Nutritional facts

Calories: 329; Fat: 27g; Saturated fat: 18g; Net Carbohydrate: 2g; Protein: 19g; Fiber: 2g;

Hamburger

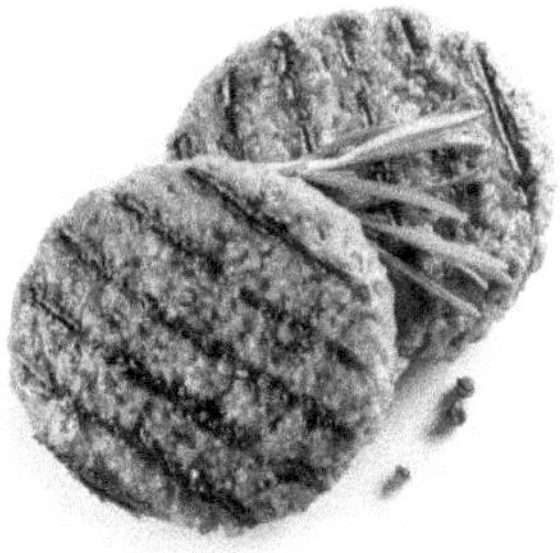

Prep time: 5 minutes, Cooking time: 10 minutes, Servings: 2

Ingredients

- Ground beef - 4/5 pound
- Salt - ¾ tsp
- Ground black pepper - ½ tsp
- Olive oil - 1 tbsp
- Lettuce leaves - 2

For Topping:

- Cooked bacon - 2½ oz
- Shredded lettuce, shredded - 1 oz
- Medium tomato, sliced - ½
- Medium red onion, sliced - ½
- Mayonnaise - 4 tbsp

Instructions

1. Place ground beef in a bowl, season with salt and black pepper, stir well and then shape into two patties.
2. Place a griddle pan over medium heat, add oil and when hot, add patties and cook for 4 to 5 minutes per side or until nicely golden brown and cooked.
3. When done, place a patty into each lettuce leaf, then top with lettuce, tomato, onion, and mayonnaise and serve.

Nutritional facts

Calories: 533; Fat: 44g; Saturated fat: 32g; Net Carbohydrate: 3g; Protein: 27g; Fiber: 5g;

Spicy Roasted Pecans

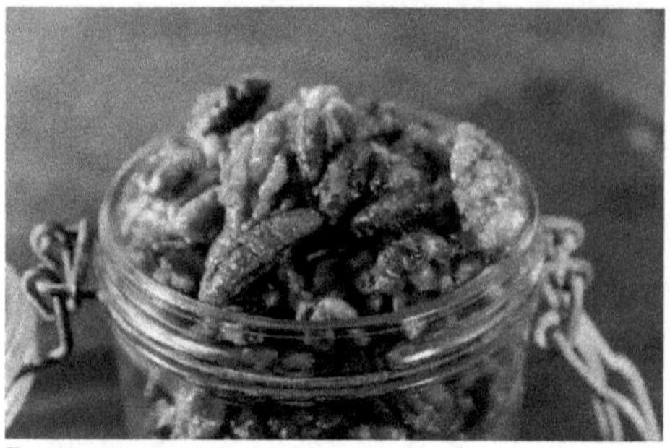

Prep time: 10 minutes, Cooking time: 5 minutes, Servings: 2

Ingredients

- Pecans – 4 oz
- Salt – ½ tsp
- Red chili powder – ½ tsp
- Ground cumin – ½ tsp
- Coconut oil – ½ tbsp

Instructions

1. Place a frying pan over medium heat, add all the ingredients in it, stir well and cook for 3 minutes or more until warm through.
2. Remove pan from heat, let pecans cool for 5 minutes and then serve.

Nutritional facts

Calories: 281; Fat: 29g; Saturated fat: 20g; Net Carbohydrate: 2g; Protein: 4g; Fiber: 4g;

Ranch Dip

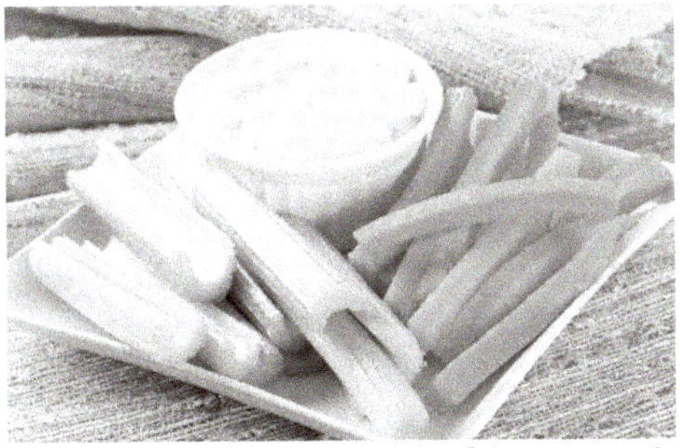

Prep time: 15 minutes, Cooking time: 0 minutes, Servings: 2

Ingredients

- Ranch seasoning – 2 tbsp
- Mayonnaise – 1 cup
- Crème Fraiche – ½ cup

Instructions

1. Place all the ingredients in a bowl, whisk until combined and let cool in the refrigerator for 15 minutes.
2. Serve dip with low-carb vegetable slices.

Nutritional facts

Calories: 241; Fat: 26g; Saturated fat: 18g; Net Carbohydrate: 1g; Protein: 1g; Fiber: 0g;

Avocado Hummus

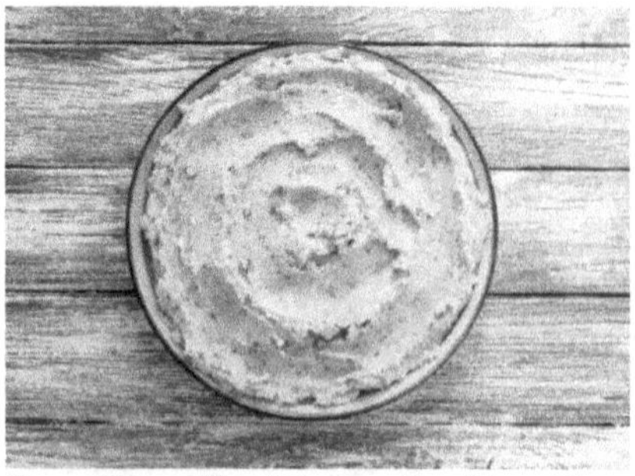

Prep time: 5 minutes, Cooking time: 0 minutes, Servings: 2

Ingredients

- Medium avocado, pitted and scooped – 1
- Chopped fresh cilantro – 2 ½ tbsp
- Minced garlic – 1/8 tsp
- Sunflower seeds – 1 ½ tbsp
- Lemon juice – 2 ½ tbsp
- Salt – 1/6 tsp
- Ground black pepper – 1/10 tsp
- Ground cumin – 1/6 tsp
- Olive oil – 2 ½ tbsp
- Tahini – 1 ½ tbsp

Instructions

1. Place avocado flesh in a blender, add remaining ingredients and pulse for 1 to 2 minutes or until smooth.
2. Tip hummus in a bowl and serve as you like.

Nutritional facts

Calories: 417; Fat: 41g; Saturated fat: 35g; Net Carbohydrate: 4g; Protein: 5g; Fiber: 8g;

Crackers

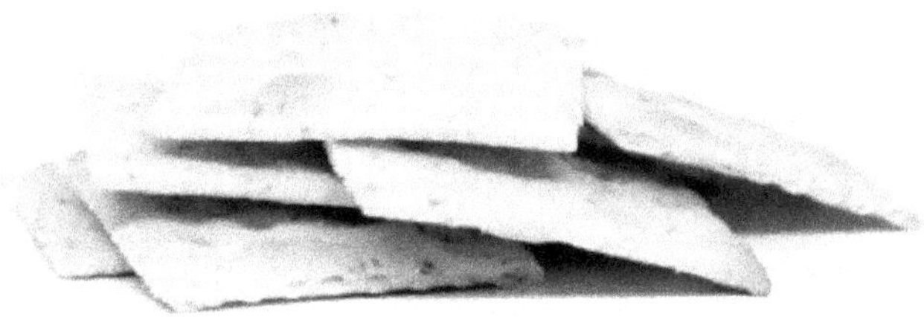

Prep time: 10 minutes, Cooking time: 11 minutes, Servings: 2

Ingredients

- Almond flour - ½ cup
- Cream cheese, soften - 1 oz
- Egg - ½
- Grated mozzarella cheese - 1 cup

Instructions

1. Set oven to 425 ° F and let preheat.
2. Meanwhile, take a large baking sheet, line it with parchment paper and set aside until required.
3. Place cream cheese and mozzarella cheese in a heatproof bowl, cover cheeses with flour and then cover the bowl with a paper towel.
4. Place the bowl into microwave and heat for 30 seconds or until cheese bubbles.
5. Then remove the bowl from heat, uncover it and stir well until a smooth dough comes together.
6. Let the dough cool for 5 minutes or more until warm to touch, then add egg and stir until incorporated.
7. Place a parchment sheet on clean working space, place dough it, then cover it with another parchment sheet and roll the dough to 1mm thickness crust by using a rolling pin.
8. Then cut out 1-inch square pieces using a pizza cutter and place the squares onto a prepared baking sheet.
9. Place the baking sheet into the oven and bake crackers for 5 minutes per side or until nicely golden and crisp, flipping the crackers halfway through.
10. When done, transfer crackers on the wire rack, let them cool and then serve with favorite Keto dip.

Nutritional facts

Calories: 52; Fat: 4g; Saturated fat: 1g; Net Carbohydrate: 1g; Protein: 3g; Fiber: 0g;

Mexican Hot Chocolate

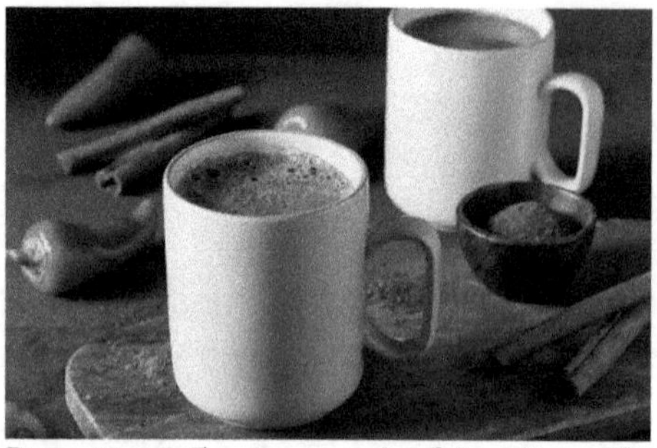

Prep time: 5 minutes, Cooking time: 5 minutes, Servings: 2

Ingredients

- Cocoa powder, unsweetened – 2 tbsp
- Chipotle powder – ¼ tsp
- Swerve sweetener – 1 tbsp
- Ground cinnamon, divided –¼ tsp
- Almond milk, unsweetened and full-fat – 1 ¼ cup
- Heavy cream – ½ cup
- Whipped cream – 2 tbsp

Instructions

1. Take a medium saucepan, place it over medium heat, add all the ingredients except for whipped cream and stir until mixed.
2. Bring the mixture to simmer and cook for 3 minutes or more until well heated.
3. Remove pan from heat, evenly pour hot chocolate between two mugs and top each mug with a tablespoon of whipped cream and sprinkle with cinnamon.
4. Serve immediately.

Nutritional facts

Calories: 433; Fat: 45g; Saturated fat: 37g; Net Carbohydrate: 2.1g; Protein: 3.4g; Fiber: 0.4g;

Mozzarella Sticks

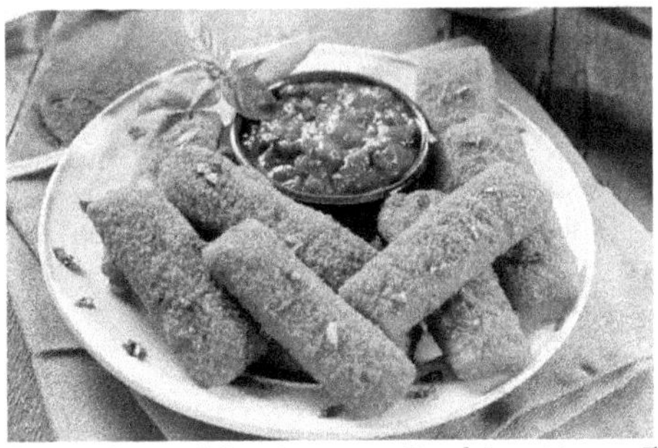

Prep time: 10 minutes, Cooking time: 5 minutes, Servings: 2

Ingredients

- Sticks of mozzarella cheese, halved – 4, each about 1 ounce
- Coconut flour – ½ tbsp
- Garlic powder – ¼ tsp
- Salt – ½ tsp
- Ground black pepper – ½ tsp
- Italian seasoning – ½ tsp
- Grated parmesan cheese – ¼ cup and ½ tbsp
- Egg – ½
- Olive oil – 1 ½ cups

Instructions

1. Crack the egg in a bowl, season with salt and black pepper and whisk until blended.
2. Place remaining ingredients in a shallow dish, except for mozzarella cheese and oil, and stir until mixed.
3. Working on one stick of cheese, first dip into the egg mixture, dredge with flour mixture, then dip into the egg again and cover with flour mixture.
4. Place coated mozzarella cheese sticks on a plate and place in freezer for 25 minutes.
5. Place a skillet pan over medium heat, grease with oil and when hot, add cheese sticks and cook for 2 minutes per side or until nicely golden brown on all sides.
6. Serve cheese sticks with a favorite dip.

Nutritional facts

Calories: 390; Fat: 28g; Saturated fat: 21g; Net Carbohydrate: 1.8g; Protein: 35g; Fiber: 1.3g;

Zucchini Chips

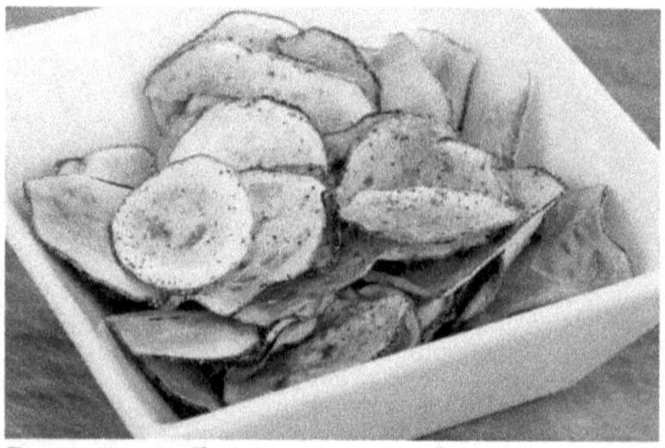

Prep time: 5 minutes, Cooking time: 3 hours, Servings: 2

Ingredients

- Zucchini, thinly sliced – 2 cups
- Sea salt – 1 tsp
- Apple cider vinegar – 1 tbsp
- Avocado oil – 1 tbsp

Instructions

1. Set oven to 200 ° F and let preheat.
2. Place olive oil and vinegar in a bowl and whisk until combined.
3. Place thinly sliced zucchini in a large bowl, drizzle with the vinegar mixture and toss until evenly coated.
4. Place zucchini chips on a baking sheet in a single layer and then bake for 2 to 3 hours or until crisp, rotating baking sheet halfway through.
5. Serve straight away.

Nutritional facts

Calories: 63 Fat: 5.1g; Saturated fat: 0.8g; Net Carbohydrate: 2.8g; Protein: 1.6g; Fiber: 1.3g;

Cream Cheese Stuffed Peppers

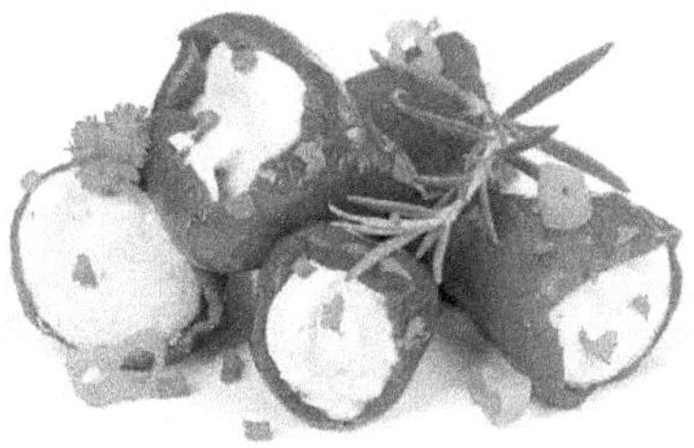

Prep time: 10 minutes, Cooking time: 20 minutes, Servings: 2

Ingredients

- Baby peppers – 6
- Cream cheese, soften – ½ cup

Instructions

1. Cut off the top from each pepper, then carefully remove seeds from the inside and then use a butter knife to stuff each pepper with cream cheese until completely full.
2. Serve immediately.

Nutritional facts

Calories: 79; Fat: 7g; Saturated fat: 3.7g; Net Carbohydrate: 1.7g; Protein: 1g; Fiber: 1.3g;

Cream Cheese Dip with Herbs

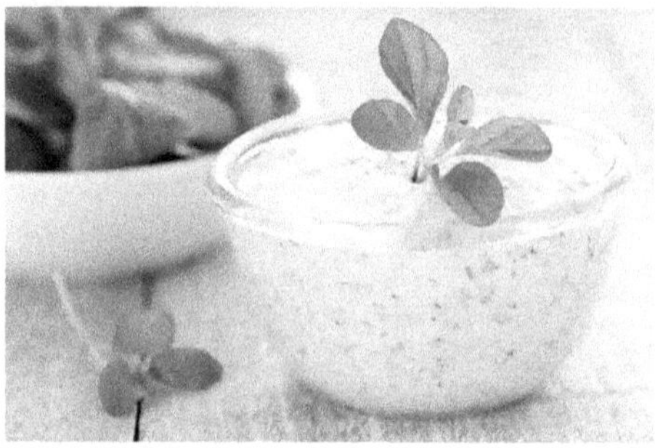

Prep time: 10 minutes, Cooking time: 5 minutes, Servings: 2

Ingredients

- Fresh parsley, chopped – 4 tbsp
- Minced garlic – ¼ tsp
- Salt – ¼ tsp
- Ground black pepper – ¼ tsp
- Lemon, zested – ¼
- Olive oil – 1 tsp
- Cream cheese – 4 oz
- Stalks of celery – 2

Instructions

1. Place all the ingredients except for celery in a bowl, stir until mixed and then chill in the refrigerator for 10 minutes.
2. Meanwhile, cut celery stalk into 2-inch pieces.
3. Serve cream cheese dip with celery pieces.

Nutritional facts

Calories: 229; Fat: 22g; Saturated fat: 14g; Net Carbohydrate: 5g; Protein: 4g; Fiber: 1g;

Chapter 5 Dinner

Rotisserie Chicken with Béarnaise Sauce

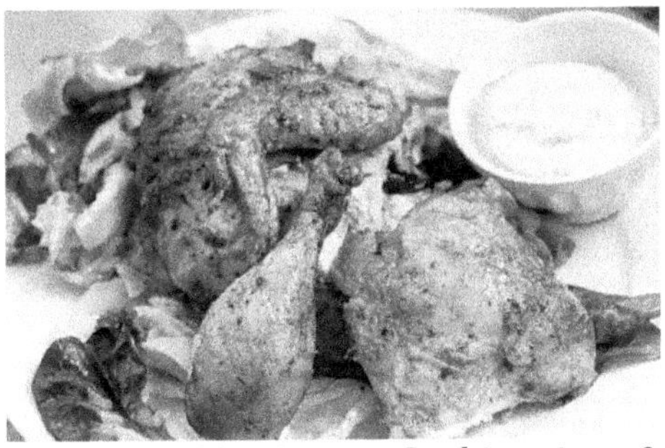

Prep time: 10 minutes, Cooking time: 0 minutes, Servings: 2

Ingredients

- Rotisserie chicken – 1
- Leafy greens – 1½ oz

For Béarnaise Sauce

- Red chili pepper, deseeded and chopped – ½
- Onion powder – ¼ tsp
- Salt – ¾ tsp
- Ground black pepper – ½ tsp
- Tomato paste – 1 tsp
- White wine vinegar – 1 tsp
- Egg yolks – 2
- Butter, melted – 51/3 oz

Instructions

1. Prepare sauce and for this, crack eggs and separate egg yolks and whites.
2. Take egg yolks and gradually beat in melted butter until smooth and thick sauce comes together.
3. Place chili in a heatproof mug, add onion powder and vinegar, stir until mixed and then add to egg yolk mixture along with tomato paste.
4. Season sauce with salt and black pepper and stir until well incorporated.
5. Cut chicken into half, divide it between two plates and serve with prepared sauce and leafy greens.

Nutritional facts

Calories: 1074; Fat: 94g; Saturated fat: 78g; Net Carbohydrate: 3g; Protein: 57g; Fiber: 1g;

Cajun Spiced Crab Casserole

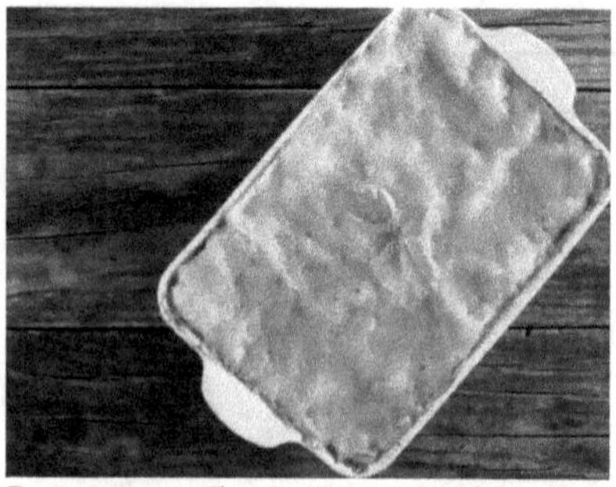

Prep time: 5 minutes, Cooking time: 35 minutes, Servings: 2

Ingredients

- Cooked crab meat – 8 oz
- Medium white onion, peeled and chopped – ½
- Celery stalks, chopped – 2½ oz
- Salt, divided – ¾ tsp
- Ground black pepper, divided – ½ tsp
- Paprika powder – 1 tsp
- Cayenne pepper – 1/8 tsp
- Shredded white cheddar cheese – 1½ cups
- Butter, for frying – 1 tbsp
- Mayonnaise – 2/3 cup
- Eggs, beaten – 2

Instructions

1. Set oven to 350 º F and let preheat.
2. Place a frying pan over medium heat, add butter and when it melts, add onion and cook for 5 minutes or more until translucent and then season with ½ teaspoon salt and ¼ teaspoon black pepper, set aside until required.
3. Crack eggs in a bowl, add crab meat, paprika, cayenne pepper, remaining salt, and black pepper and 1 cup cheese, then add onion mixture and stir until combined.
4. Spoon the mixture into a baking dish, spread evenly and then top with cheese.
5. Place the baking sheet into the oven and bake for 30 minutes or until the top is nicely golden brown.
6. Serve straight away.

Nutritional facts

Calories: 1107; Fat: 98g; Saturated fat: 83g; Net Carbohydrate: 6g; Protein: 47g; Fiber: 2g;

Turkey with Cream-Cheese Sauce

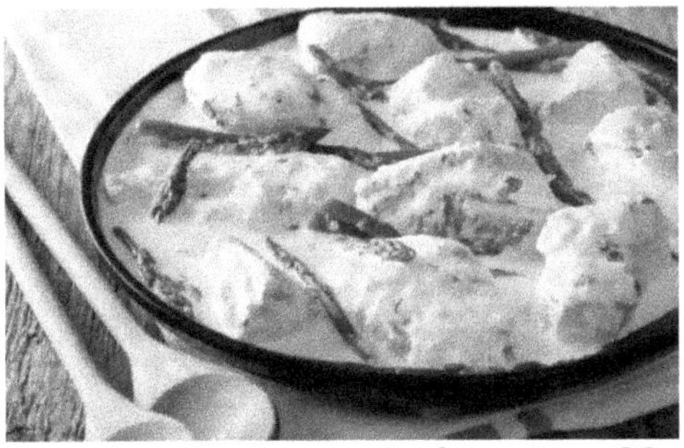

Prep time: 5 minutes, Cooking time: 23 minutes, Servings: 2

Ingredients

- Turkey breast - 10 oz
- Small capers - 1/6 cup
- Salt - ¾ tsp
- Ground black pepper - ¾ tsp
- Soy sauce - ½ tbsp
- Butter - 1 tbsp
- Crème Fraiche - 1 cup
- Cream cheese - 3½ oz

Instructions

1. Set 350 ° F and let preheat.
2. Place a heatproof frying pan over medium heat, add ½ tablespoon butter and when it melts, add turkey and season with a ½ teaspoon each of salt and black pepper.
3. Cook turkey for 5 minutes or until nicely golden brown on all side, then transfer frying pan into the oven and cook for 7 to 10 minutes or until a meat thermometer inserted in turkey reads 165 ° F.
4. When done, transfer turkey to a plate and cover with aluminum foil, set aside until required.
5. Pour turkey drippings from the frying pan into a small saucepan, add crème Fraiche and cream cheese, stir well and bring the mixture to boil over medium heat.
6. Then switch heat to low heat and simmer sauce for 3 to 5 minutes or until thickened.
7. Season sauce with salt and black pepper and remove the pan from heat, set aside until required.
8. Return frying pan over medium heat, add remaining butter and when it melts, add capers, and fry got 2 to 3 minutes or until crispy.
9. Serve turkey with prepared sauce and top with fried capers.

Nutritional facts

Calories: 793; Fat: 67g; Saturated fat: 53g; Net Carbohydrate: 7g; Protein: 43g; Fiber: 0g;

Red Pesto Pork Chops

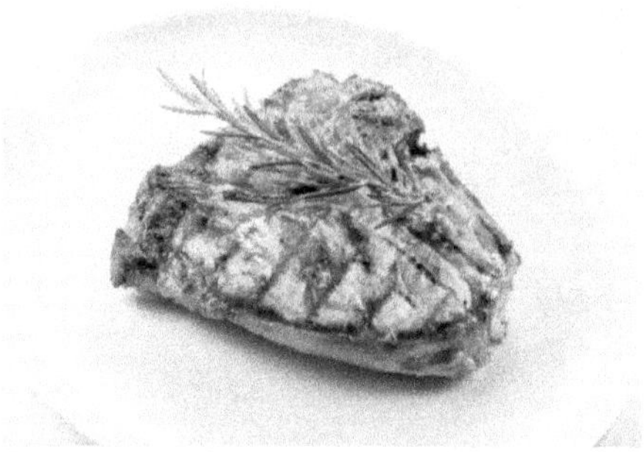

Prep time: 5 minutes, Cooking time: 15 minutes, Servings: 2

Ingredients

- Pork chops – 2
- Salt – ½ tsp
- Ground black pepper – ½ tsp
- Butter – 1 tbsp
- Red pesto, divided – 3 tbsp
- Mayonnaise – 5 tbsp

Instructions

1. Brush pork chops with 2 tablespoons red pesto and season with salt and black pepper.
2. Place a frying pan over medium heat, add butter and when it melts, add chops and cook for 9 minutes.
3. Then reduce heat to low heat and simmer pork chops for 5 minutes.
4. Meanwhile, place mayonnaise in a bowl, add remaining pesto and whisk until combined.
5. Serve pork chops with pesto mayonnaise.

Nutritional facts

Calories: 448; Fat: 61g; Saturated fat: 3g; Net Carbohydrate: 5.4g; Protein: 37.5g; Fiber: 0.6g;

Baked Salmon with Pesto

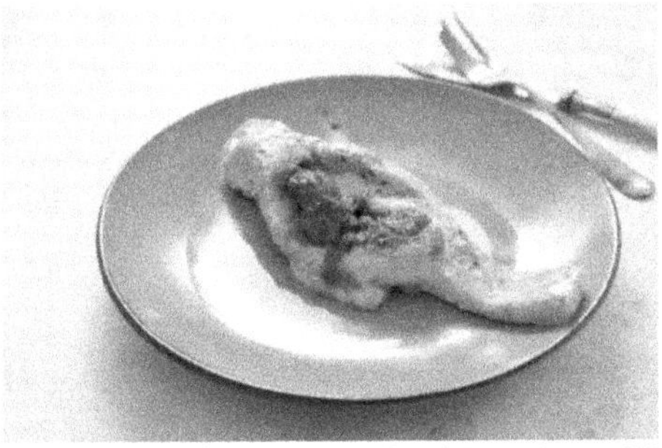

Prep time: 5 minutes, Cooking time: 30 minutes, Servings: 2

Ingredients

- Salmon fillet - 15 oz
- Salt - ¾ tsp
- Ground black pepper - ½ tsp
- Green pesto - 2 tbsp

Green sauce

- Green pesto - 1 oz
- Salt - ½ tsp
- Ground black pepper - ½ tsp
- Mayonnaise - ½ cup
- Greek yogurt - 4 tbsp

Instructions

1. Set oven to 400 ° F and let preheat.
2. Place pesto on top of salmon, spread evenly and then season with salt and black pepper.
3. Place salmon on a baking sheet, then place it in an oven and bake for 30 minutes or until salmon is cooked through.
4. Meanwhile, prepare the green sauce and for this, place all the ingredients for sauce and whisk until combined.
5. Serve salmon with green sauce.

Nutritional facts

Calories: 1030; Fat: 90g; Saturated fat: 76g; Net Carbohydrate: 3g; Protein: 49g; Fiber: 0g;

Bacon-Wrapped Meatloaf

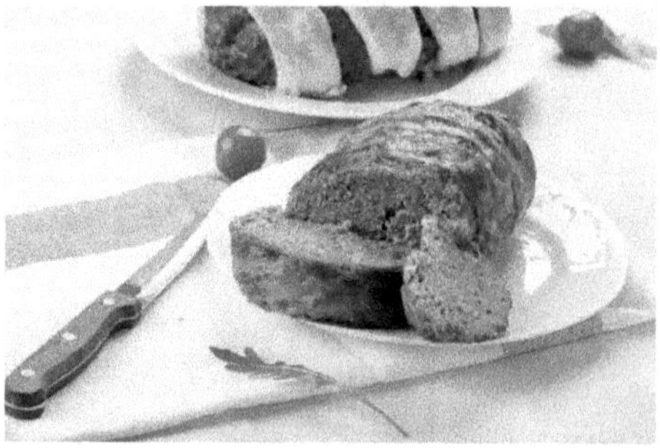

Prep time: 5 minutes, Cooking time: 50 minutes, Servings: 2

Ingredients

- Sliced bacon – 3½ oz
- Ground beef – 12 oz
- Medium white onion, peeled and chopped – ½
- Salt – ½ tsp
- Ground black pepper – ¼ tsp
- Dried basil – ½ tbsp
- Butter – 1 tbsp
- Egg – ½
- Heavy whipping cream, divided – 2/3 cup, and 4 tbsp
- Shredded cheddar cheese – ¼ cup

Instructions

1. Set oven to 400 ° F and let preheat.
2. Meanwhile, place a frying pan over medium heat, add butter and when it melts, add onion and cook for 3 minutes until soft and golden.
3. Spoon the onion in a large bowl, add remaining ingredients except for bacon and 2/3 cup of cream, and mix until well combined.
4. Shape mixture into a loaf, then place it in a baking dish and wrap loaf in bacon slices.
5. Place baking dish into the oven and bake for 45 minutes, cover meatloaf with aluminum foil after 30 minutes or baking.
6. When done, transfer meatloaf to a cutting board and pour the juices into a small saucepan.
7. Add remaining heavy cream, whisk until combined, then place the pan over low heat, bring to boil and simmer the sauce for 10 to 15 minutes or until sauce reduce to desired thickness.
8. Cut meatloaf into slices and serve with prepared sauce.

Nutritional facts

Calories: 1038; Fat: 90g; Saturated fat: 79g; Net Carbohydrate: 6g; Protein: 48g; Fiber: 1g;

Lamb Chops with Herb Butter

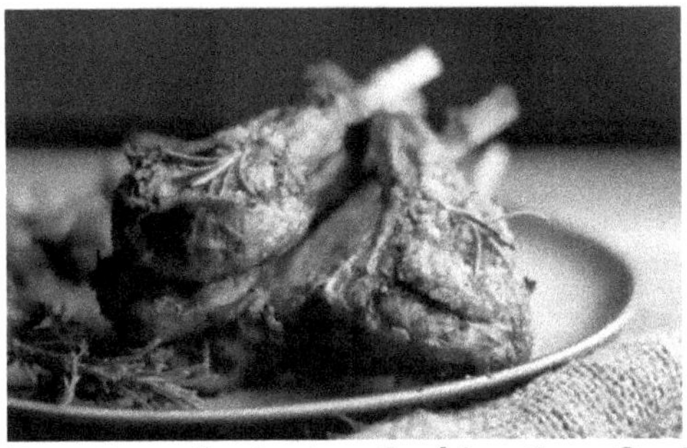

Prep time: 5 minutes, Cooking time: 8 minutes, Servings: 2

Ingredients

- Lamb chops - 4
- Salt - ¾ tsp
- Ground black pepper - ½ tsp
- Butter - ½ tbsp
- Olive oil - ½ tbsp

For Serving

- Herb butter - 2 oz
- Lemon, cut into wedges - ½

Instructions

1. Place a frying pan over medium heat, add butter and oil, and let heat.
2. Season pork chops with salt and black pepper, add them into the frying pan and cook for 3 to 4 minutes per side or until nicely golden brown and cooked.
3. Serve pork chops with herb butter and lemon wedges.

Nutritional facts

Calories: 729; Fat: 62g; Saturated fat: 49g; Net Carbohydrate: 0.3g; Protein: 43g; Fiber: 0g;

Cuban Roast Pork

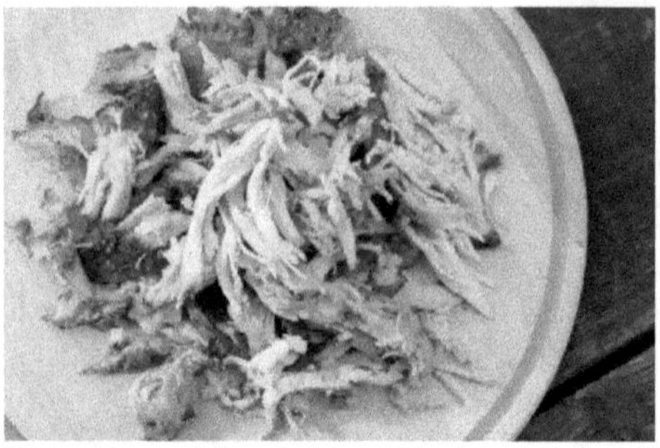

Prep time: 10 minutes, Cooking time: 8 hours and 35 minutes, Servings: 2

Ingredients

- Pork shoulder, boneless and fat trimmed - 1½ pound
- Large red onion, peeled and diced - 1/3
- Minced garlic - 1 tsp
- Salt - 1 1/3 tsp
- Ground black pepper - 1/3 tsp
- Ground cumin - 2/3 tsp
- Fresh oregano - 2/3 tbsp
- Olive oil - 1 ½ tbsp
- Lemon, juiced - 1 ¼ tbsp
- Orange juice - 3 tbsp

Instructions

1. Place pork shoulder in a shallow dish, season with salt and set aside.
2. Place remaining ingredients in a food processor, pulse for 1 minute or until smooth, then pour this mixture all over the pork shoulder and massage it into the pork.
3. Cover the dish and marinate the pork in the refrigerator for 8 hours, turning pork halfway through in the marinade.
4. Then remove pork from the refrigerator and let sit at room temperature for 1 hour.
5. Plugin and switch on the slow cooker, place marinated pork in it, fat-side up, then shut with lid and cook for 8 hours at low heat setting until done.
6. Then transfer pork to a sheet pan and roast it for 30 minutes or until crispy and nicely golden brown.
7. Meanwhile, pour the juices from the slow cooker in a saucepan and cook for 3 to 5 minutes or until sauce is reduced by half.
8. When pork is ready, shred it with two forms, pour in the sauce and toss until mixed.
9. Serve straight away.

Nutritional facts

Calories: 912; Fat: 70g; Saturated fat: 57g; Net Carbohydrate: 6g; Protein: 59g; Fiber: 2g;

Loaded Cauliflower

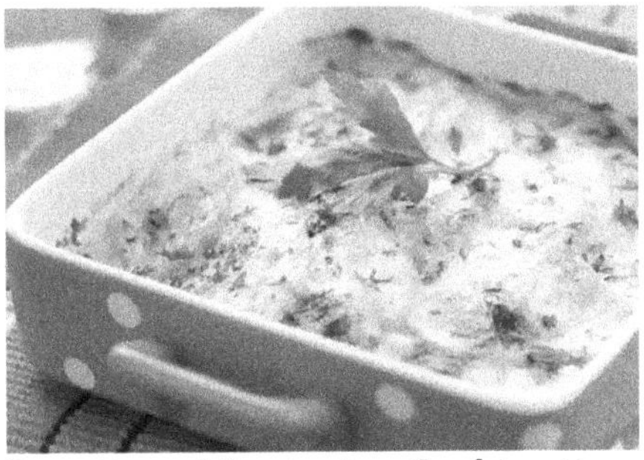

Prep time: 10 minutes, Cooking time: 8 minutes, Servings: 2

Ingredients

- Cooked bacon, crumbled - 1 slice
- Cauliflower florets - 1/3 pound
- Snipped chives - 2/3 tbsp
- Salt - ¼ tsp
- Ground black pepper - 1/8 tsp
- Garlic powder - 1/8 tsp
- Butter - 1 tbsp
- Sour cream - 1 1/3 ounces
- Grated cheddar cheese - 1/3 cup
- Water - 2 tbsp

Instructions

1. Place cauliflower florets in a heatproof bowl, add water, then cover the bowl with plastic wrap and microwave for 5 to 8 minutes or until florets are tender and cooked.
2. Uncover the bowl, then drain florets and let sit for 2 minutes.
3. Then transfer florets into a food processor and pulse for 1 minute or more until fluffy.
4. Add butter, garlic, and sour cream and blend for 1 minute or more until mashed.
5. Tip mashed cauliflower in a casserole, add half of the cheddar cheese, most of the chives, salt and black pepper and stir until combined.
6. Top cauliflower with remaining cheddar cheese, place casserole under the heated broiler and then cook for 3 minutes or more until the top is nicely golden brown.
7. Top cauliflower with bacon and chives and serve.

Nutritional facts

Calories: 199; Fat: 17g; Saturated fat: 10g; Net Carbohydrate: 3g; Protein: 8g; Fiber: 2g;

Garlic Butter Steak

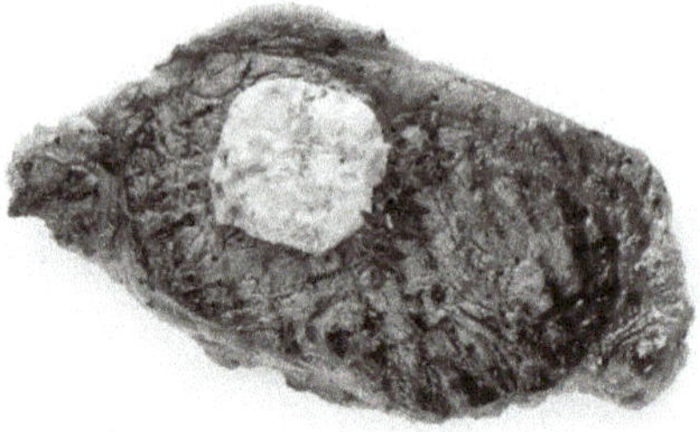

Prep time: 10 minutes, Cooking time: 6 minutes, Servings: 2

Ingredients

- Steak, cut into 4 pieces – ¾ pound
- Minced garlic – 1 ½ tsp
- Salt – 1 tsp
- Ground black pepper – ¾ tsp
- Olive oil – 1 tbsp
- Butter – 2 tbsp
- Chopped parsley – ½ tbsp

Instructions

1. Season steaks with salt and black pepper until evenly coated.
2. Place a skillet pan over medium-high heat, add oil and when hot, add seasoned steaks and cook for 3 minutes per side or more until cooked to desired doneness.
3. When done, transfer steaks to a plate and let rest for 5 minutes.
4. Meanwhile, place a skillet pan over low heat, add garlic, season with 1/8 teaspoon salt and cook for 4 minutes or until nicely golden.
5. Slice steaks across the grain and evenly divide between two plates.
6. Drizzle steaks with prepared garlic mixture, then sprinkle with parsley and serve.

Nutritional facts

Calories: 429; Fat: 31g; Saturated fat: 18g; Net Carbohydrate: 1g; Protein: 37g; Fiber: 1g;

Garlic Scallops

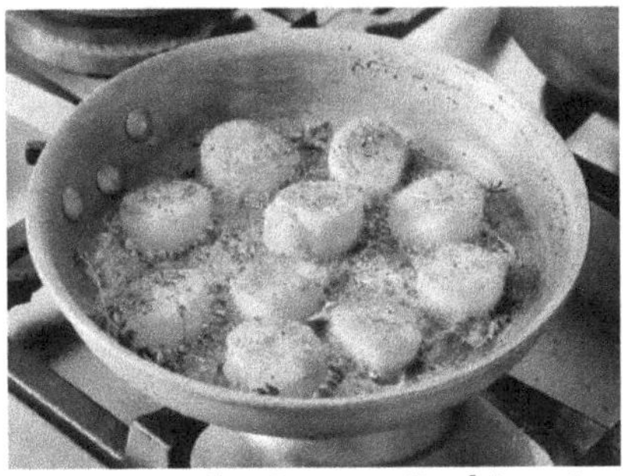

Prep time: 5 minutes, Cooking time: 10 minutes, Servings: 2

Ingredients

- Large scallops – 1 pound
- Chopped parsley – ¼ cup
- Minced garlic – 2 tsp
- Large lemon, juiced and zested – 1
- Sea salt – ½ tsp
- Ground black pepper – ¼ tsp
- Red pepper flakes – ¼ tsp
- Clarified butter – ¼ cup
- Olive oil – 1 tsp

Instructions

1. Pat dry scallops, then place them in a bowl, season with salt, black pepper, red pepper flakes, then drizzle with clarified butter and toss until evenly coated.
2. Place a skillet pan over medium heat, grease its bottom with oil, then add scallops in a single layer and cook for 2 minutes per side or until nicely golden.
3. Cook remaining scallops in the same manner, then return all scallops into the pan, add garlic, stir until mixed and remove the pan from heat.
4. Let scallops rest in pan for 1 minute, then drizzle with lemon juice and olive oil, and then sprinkle with lemon zest and parsley.
5. Serve straight away.

Nutritional facts

Calories: 391; Fat: 26g; Saturated fat: 15g; Net Carbohydrate: 0g; Protein: 28g; Fiber: 0g;

Mozzarella Chicken

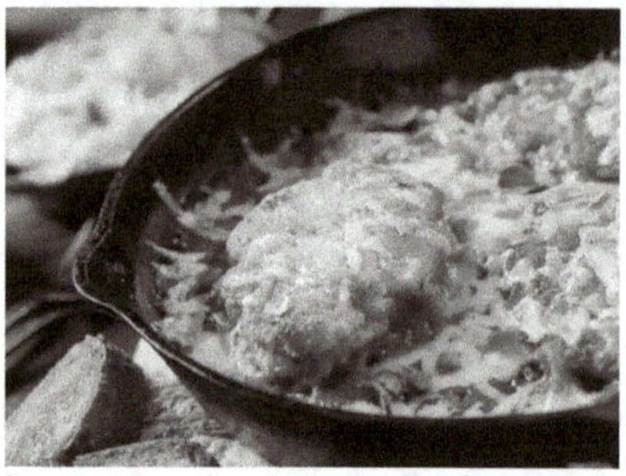

Prep time: 2 minutes, Cooking time: 20 minutes, Servings: 2

Ingredients

- Small chicken breasts - 2
- Chopped white onions - ¼ cup
- Crushed tomatoes - 7 ounce
- Minced garlic - ½ tbsp
- Salt - ¼ tsp
- Ground black pepper - ¼ tsp
- Red pepper flakes - ¼ tsp
- Dried basil - 1/8 teaspoon
- Italian seasoning - ¼ tsp
- Sun-dried tomato pesto - ½ tbsp
- Olive oil, divided - 1 tbsp
- Shredded mozzarella cheese - ½ cup
- Water - 3 tbsp

Instructions

1. Season chicken with a ¼ teaspoon each of salt and black pepper until evenly coated on both side.
2. Place a skillet pan over medium-high heat, add ½ tablespoon oil and when hot, add seasoned chicken and cook for 3 to 5 minutes per side or until nicely golden brown and cooked through, set aside until required and keep chicken warm.
3. Prepare a tomato sauce and for this, switch on broiler and let preheat.
4. Return skillet pan over medium heat, add remaining oil and when hot, add onion and cook for 2 to 3 minutes or until softened.
5. Add garlic, cook for 30 seconds or until fragrant, then add tomatoes along with remaining ingredients except for cheese and water, and stir until combined.
6. Simmer sauce, then pour in water, switch heat to a low level and simmer the sauce for 5 minutes or until slightly thick, covering the pan.
7. Then add chicken into tomato sauce, spoon some of the sauce on chicken and then top the chicken with cheese.
8. Transfer pan into the broiler and cook chicken for 2 minutes until cheese melts and the top is nicely golden.
9. Serve straight away.

Nutritional facts

Calories: 385; Fat: 25.4g; Saturated fat: 7.9g; Net Carbohydrate: 2.2g; Protein: 31.7g; Fiber: 1.8g;

Fish Fingers with Mayo Dip

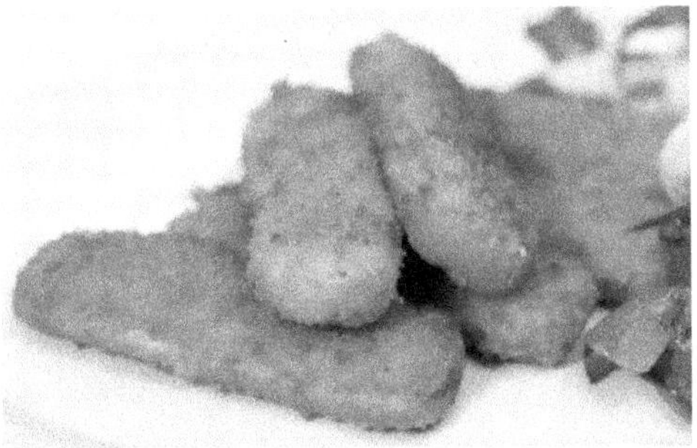

Prep time: 5 minutes, Cooking time: 13 minutes, Servings: 2

Ingredients

- Almond flour– 1/3 cup
- Cod, cut into slices – 8.8 oz
- Onion powder – ½ tsp
- Garlic powder – ¼ tsp
- Sea salt – ½ tsp
- Paprika – ¼ tsp
- Egg, beaten – 1

Mayo Dip:

- Small red chili pepper, deseeded – 1
- Minced garlic – 2 tsp
- Fresh parsley – 2.1 oz
- Fresh oregano – ¼ cup
- Salt – ½ tsp
- Ground black pepper – ½ tsp
- Apple cider vinegar – 2 tbsp
- Olive oil – ½ cup
- Mayonnaise – ¼ cup

Instructions

1. Set oven to 410 ° F and let preheat.
2. Prepare fish and for this, crack an egg in a bowl and beat it slightly.
3. Place remaining ingredients in a shallow dish and stir until mixed.
4. Cut cod into 1-inch fingers, then dip each fish finger into the egg, dredge in almond flour mixture until evenly coated and then place on a greased baking tray.
5. Place the baking tray into the oven, then bake for 8 minutes, flip the fish finger and continue baking for 5 minutes or until nicely golden brown.
6. Meanwhile, prepare mayonnaise dip and for this, place all the ingredients for the dip in a bowl and whisk until well combined.
7. Serve fish fingers with mayonnaise dip.

Nutritional facts

Calories: 505; Fat: 40.1g; Saturated fat: 33.6g; Net Carbohydrate: 3g; Protein: 29.6g; Fiber: 2.3g;

Butter Cod

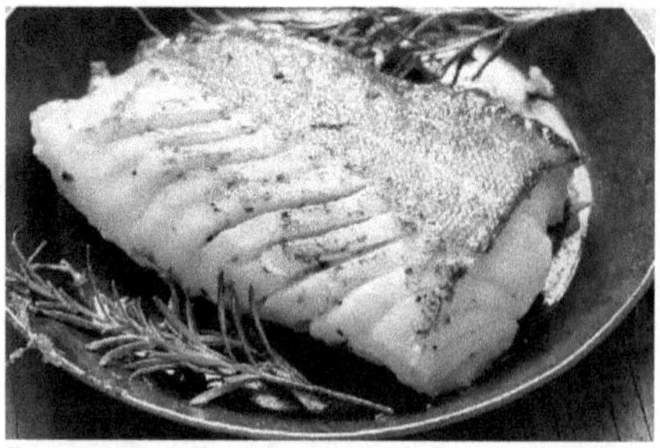

Prep time: 5 minutes, Cooking time: 6 minutes, Servings: 2

Ingredients

For Cod:

- Cod fillets - ¾ pound
- Butter, sliced - 3 tbsp
- Chopped parsley - 1 tsp
- Lemon slices - 2

For Seasoning:

- Garlic powder - 1/8 tsp
- Salt - ¼ tsp
- Ground black pepper - 1/8 tsp
- Ground paprika - 1/3 tsp
- Dried parsley - ¼ tsp

Instructions

1. Place all the ingredients for seasoning in a small bowl and stir until mixed.
2. Cut fish into bite-size pieces and then sprinkle with prepared seasoning until evenly coated.
3. Place a skillet pan over medium-high heat, add 1 ½ tablespoon butter and when it melts, add seasoned cod and cook for 2 minutes.
4. Switch heat to medium heat, turn the cod, then top with remaining butter and continue cooking for 4 minutes or until butter melts and cod is cooked through.
5. Then remove the pan from heat, sprinkle cod with parsley and serve with lemon slices.

Nutritional facts

Calories: 294; Fat: 18g; Saturated fat: 11g; Net Carbohydrate: 1g; Protein: 30g; Fiber: 0g;

Cashew Chicken

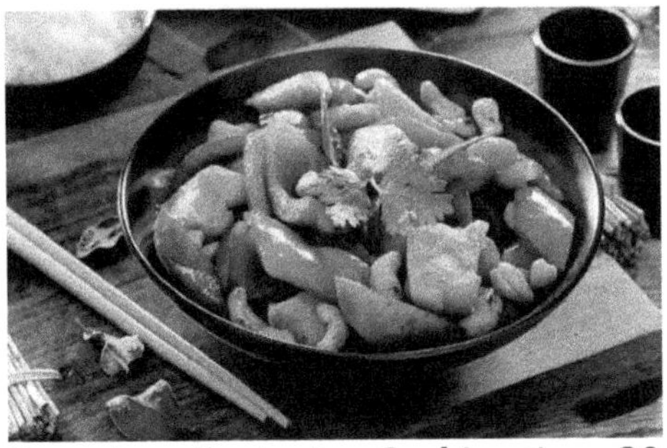

Prep time: 5 minutes, Cooking time: 20 minutes, Servings: 2

Ingredients

- Boneless chicken thighs, cut into chunks – 2
- Green onions, chopped – 1 tbsp
- Medium white onion, peeled and cut into chunks – ¼
- Medium green bell pepper, cut into chunks – ½
- Minced garlic – 1 tbsp
- Grated ginger – ½ tsp
- Salt – ½ tsp
- Ground black pepper – ¼ tsp
- Cashews – ¼ cup
- Sesame seeds – 1 tbsp
- Liquid aminos – 1 ½ tbsp
- Apple cider vinegar – 1 tbsp
- Coconut oil – 2 tbsp
- Sesame oil – 1 tbsp
- Chili garlic sauce – ½ tbsp

Instructions

1. Place a skillet pan over low heat and when hot, add cashews and cook for 8 minutes or until fragrant and nicely golden, set aside until required.
2. Return pan over high heat, add coconut oil and when hot, add chicken pieces and cook for 5 minutes or until cooked.
3. Then add onion and bell pepper pieces along with garlic and ginger, season with salt and black pepper, add chili garlic sauce and toss until combined.
4. Cook chicken and vegetables for 2 to 3 minutes, then add cashews along with vinegar and liquid aminos and continue cooking for 3 minutes or more until cooking sauce is slightly thick.
5. Remove pan from heat, drizzle sesame oil over the chicken, then sprinkle with sesame seeds and serve.

Nutritional facts

Calories: 333.3; Fat: 24g; Saturated fat: 18g; Net Carbohydrate: 6.7g; Protein: 22.6g; Fiber: 1.3g;

Chapter 6 Dessert

Peanut Butter Cups

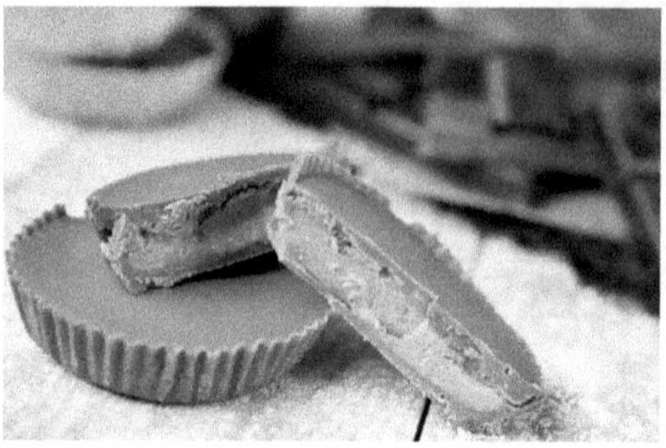

Prep time: 60 minutes, Cooking time: 8 minutes, Servings: 2

Ingredients

- Raspberries – 2 tbsp
- Water – ¾ tbsp
- Swerve Sweetener, divided – 1 1/3 tbsp
- Gelatin, grass-fed – ¼ tsp
- Creamy peanut butter – 2 tbsp
- Coconut oil – 2 tbsp

Instructions

1. Place a saucepan over medium heat, add raspberries, then pour in water and bring the mixture to boil.
2. When the mixture comes to boil, reduce heat to a low level and simmer the mixture for 5 minutes, and then mash berries with a fork.
3. Remove saucepan from heat, stir in ¾ tablespoon sweetener, and then whisk in gelatin until combined, set aside until required.
4. Take a heatproof bowl, add peanut butter and oil and stir until combined.
5. Place the bowl into the microwave, cook for 30 to 60 seconds at high heat setting or until butter melts and then stir in remaining sweetener.
6. Take two muffin cups, line them with paper liners, and then evenly spoon in prepared peanut butter mixture.
7. Place muffin cups into freezer for 15 to 30 minutes or more until firm, then top with the raspberry mixture and freeze more for 30 minutes or until set and firm.
8. Serve when ready.

Nutritional facts

Calories: 223; Fat: 21.7g; Saturated fat: 15.8g; Net Carbohydrate: 3.2g; Protein: 3.8g; Fiber: 1.3g;

Chocolate Coconut Cups

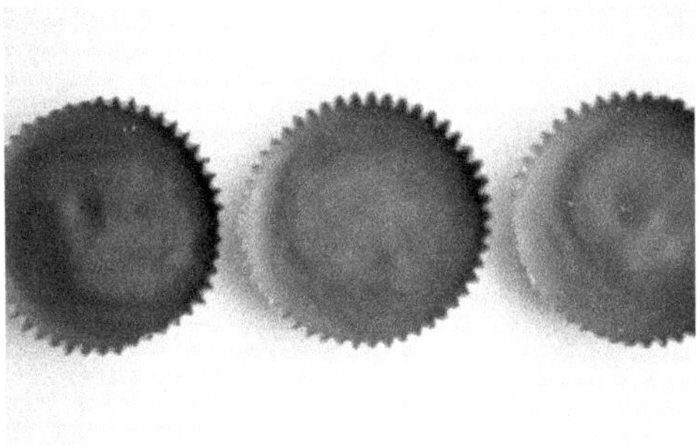

Prep time: 35 minutes, Cooking time: 5 minutes, Servings: 2

Ingredients

For Coconut Candies:

- Coconut butter - ¾ tbsp
- Coconut oil - ¾ tbsp
- Shredded coconut, unsweetened - ¾ tbsp
- Swerve sweetener - 1/3 tbsp

For Chocolate Topping:

- Chocolate, unsweetened - ¼ tbsp
- Cocoa butter, divided - 1 ¼ tbsp
- Swerve sweetener - ½ tbsp
- Cocoa powder, unsweetened - ½ tbsp
- Vanilla extract, unsweetened - 0.03 tsp

Instructions

1. Prepare coconut candies and for this, place a small saucepan over low heat, add coconut butter and oil, stir well and cook for 2 to 3 minutes or until butter melts.
2. Then stir in coconut and swerve sweetener until combined and remove the pan from heat.
3. Take two mini muffin cups, line them with a paper liner, then evenly spoon in coconut butter mixture and place them in the freezer for 30 minutes or until firm.
4. Meanwhile, prepare the chocolate topping and for this, place chocolate in a heatproof bowl, add cocoa butter and microwave for 30 to 60 seconds at high heat setting or until butter melts.
5. Add vanilla extra into cocoa butter, whisk well, then evenly spoon over firmed coconut candies and let rest for 15 minutes.
6. Serve straight away.

Nutritional facts

Calories: 240; Fat: 25g; Saturated fat: 16g; Net Carbohydrate: 1g; Protein: 2g; Fiber: 4g;

Dark Chocolate Covered Walnuts

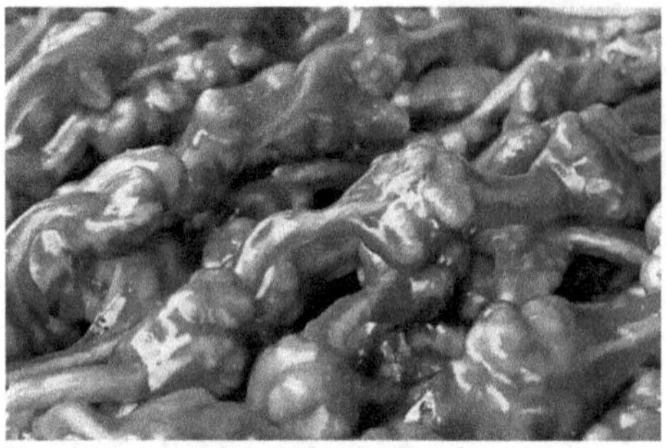

Prep time: 40 minutes, Cooking time: 3 minutes, Servings: 2

Ingredients

- Chocolate, unsweetened and chopped – 4 oz
- Swerve sweetener – ¼ cup
- Walnut oil – 3 tbsp
- Cocoa powder unsweetened – 1 tbsp
- Vanilla extract, unsweetened – ½ tsp
- Walnuts, shelled – 2 cups

Instructions

1. Place a small saucepan over low heat, add chocolate, sweetener, and oil, stir well and cook for 2 to 3 minutes or until smooth mixture comes together.
2. Remove pan from heat, add cocoa and vanilla, stir well until smooth and let cool for 5 minutes or until slightly thickened.
3. Add half of the walnuts, stir until coated, then lift out each walnut with a fork and place on a baking sheet lined with parchment paper.
4. Add remaining walnuts into chocolate mixture, stir until evenly coated, then lift out each walnut with a fork and place on a baking sheet.
5. Place the baking sheet into the freezer and chill for 30 minutes or more until firm.
6. Serve walnuts when ready.

Nutritional facts

Calories: 196; Fat: 18g; Saturated fat: 6g; Net Carbohydrate: 2g; Protein: 3g; Fiber: 3g;

Vanilla Ice Cream

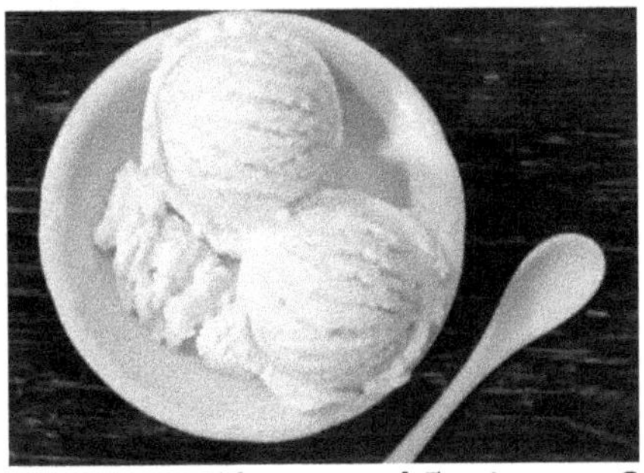

Prep time: 5 hours and 5 minutes, Cooking time: 0 minutes, Servings: 2

Ingredients

- Coconut milk, chilled – 7.5 oz.
- Heavy cream – ½ cup
- Swerve sweetener, powdered – 1 tbsp
- Vanilla extract, unsweetened – 1 tsp

Instructions

1. Transfer cream from chilled coconut milk into a bowl and blend until creamy, set aside until required.
2. Place cream in another bowl, beat at high speed until soft peaks form and then beat in sweetener and vanilla until combined.
3. Fold in coconut cream mixture and spoon the mixture into a freezer-proof bowl.
4. Place the bowl into the freezer and chill for 5 hours or until solid.
5. Serve straight away.

Nutritional facts

Calories: 127.1; Fat: 11.5g; Saturated fat: 7.3g; Net Carbohydrate: 1.8g; Protein: 1.1g; Fiber: 0.1g;

Chocolate Mug Cake

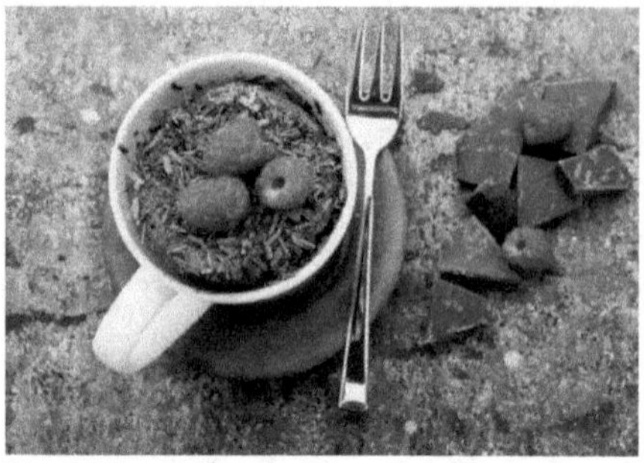

Prep time: 5 minutes, Cooking time: 3 minutes, Servings: 2

Ingredients

- Almond flour – ½ cup
- Salt – 1/8 teaspoon
- Swerve sweetener – 2 tsp
- Cocoa powder, unsweetened – 4 tbsp
- Chocolate chips, low-carb – 4 tbsp
- Baking powder – 1 tsp
- Butter – 4 tbsp
- Eggs, beaten – 2
- Whipped cream, for serving – ½ cup

Instructions

1. Take two heatproof mugs, evenly divide the butter in them and microwave for 30 seconds or until butter melts.
2. Then evenly remaining ingredients into each cup and stir until combined.
3. Return the cups into the microwave and heat for 1 minute or until cake is set.
4. Top mug cake with whipped cream and serve.

Nutritional facts

Calories: 272; Fat: 23g; Saturated fat: 17g; Net Carbohydrate: 3g; Protein: 9g; Fiber: 4g;

Lemon Curd

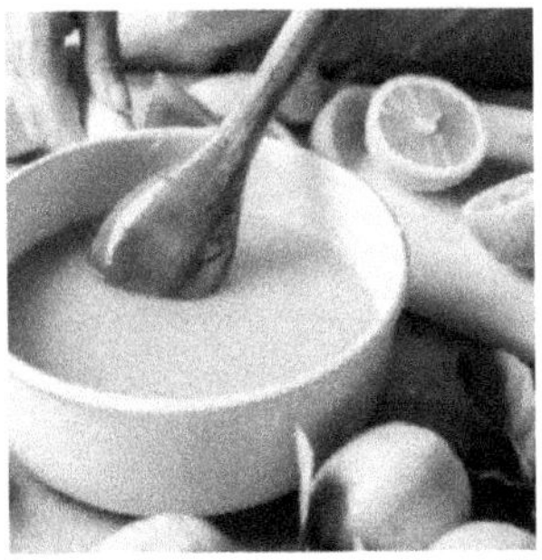

Prep time: 10 minutes, Cooking time: 12 minutes, Servings: 2

Ingredients

- Erythritol sweetener - ¼ cup
- Butter - 3 1/3 tbsp
- Lemons, juiced and zested – 2
- Eggs, small - 2
- Egg yolk - 1

Instructions

1. Take a heatproof bowl, add erythritol, butter, lemon zest, and lemon juice and whisk until just mixed.
2. Place the bowl into microwave and heat for 30 to 60 seconds or more until butter melts and then whisk well.
3. Whisk in eggs and egg yolks, then place the bowl over a saucepan containing simmering water and continue whisking for 10 minutes until the mixture coats the back of a spoon.
4. Then remove the bowl from the pan and divide evenly between sterilized jars and store them into the refrigerator to chill.
5. Serve when ready.

Nutritional facts

Calories: 258; Fat: 25g; Saturated fat: 18g; Net Carbohydrate: 2g; Protein: 7g; Fiber: 0.2g;

Chocolate Gelato

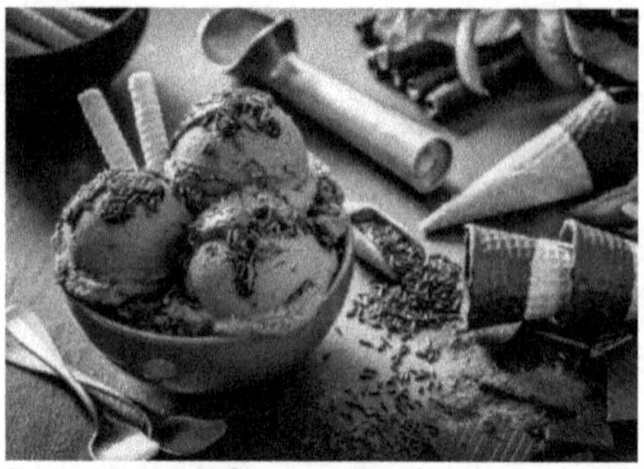

Prep time: 4 hours, Cooking time: 15 minutes, Servings: 2

Ingredients

- Heavy whipping cream – ½ cup
- Erythritol sweetener, powdered – 3 tbsp
- Cocoa powder, unsweetened – ¾ tbsp
- Egg yolk – 1
- Vanilla extract, unsweetened – ¼ tsp

Instructions

1. Place a saucepan over medium-high heat, add cream and sweetener, stir until mixed and bring the mixture to boil.
2. Reduce heat to medium-low level, simmer the mixture and then whisk in cocoa powder until well combined, stirring continuously until the mixture starts to thicken.
3. Then remove the pan from heat and cool for 5 minutes.
4. Meanwhile, place the egg yolk in a bowl, add vanilla and whisk until combined, then add into the cooled cream mixture and beat until smooth and frothy.
5. Transfer mixture into a freezer-proof bowl and chill in the freezer for 4 hours or more until set, stirring every hour.
6. Serve when ready.

Nutritional facts

Calories: 231; Fat: 22.5g; Saturated fat: 3g; Net Carbohydrate: 4.75g; Protein: 1.75g; Fiber: 0.75g;

Mint Chocolate Chip Ice Cream

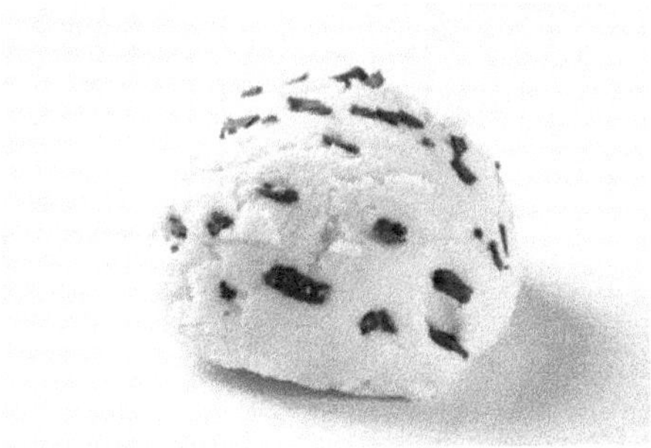

Prep time: 2 hours and 5 minutes, Cooking time: 0 minutes, Servings: 2

Ingredients

- Medium avocado, pitted and scooped – ½
- Vanilla extract – ½ tsp
- Peppermint extract – ¾ tsp
- Coconut milk, unsweetened – ½ cup
- Lemon juice – ½ tsp
- Swerve sweetener, powdered – 4 tbsp
- Chocolate chips – 1.5 ounces

Instructions

1. Place avocado in a blender, add vanilla and peppermint extract, pour in coconut milk and pulse for 1 to 2 minutes or until smooth.
2. Pour the mixture into a freezer-proof container, shut with lid and place in freezer for 2 hours or more until set.
3. When ready, scoop out ice cream into bowls and serve.

Nutritional facts

Calories: 151; Fat: 15g; Saturated fat: 11g; Net Carbohydrate: 2.5g; Protein: 1.5g; Fiber: 2g;

Lime Pudding

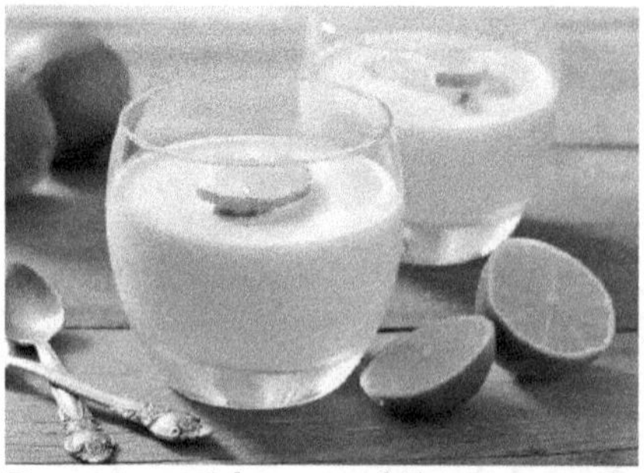

Prep time: 1 hour and 5 minutes, Cooking time: 10 minutes, Servings: 2

Ingredients

For Pudding:

- Medium avocados, pitted and scooped – 2
- Salt – 1/16 tsp
- Erythritol Syrup – 2/3 cup
- Almond extract – 2 tbsp
- Lime Juice – 1.6 oz
- Coconut Oil, melted – 3 tbsp

For Erythritol Syrup:

- boiling water – 1 cup
- erythritol sweetener – ¾ cup
- vanilla extract – 1 tsp
- Stevia – 6 drops
- Xanthan Gum powder – ¼ tsp

Instructions

1. Prepare syrup and for this, place a small pot over medium-low heat, then pour in water and add sweetener, vanilla, and stevia, stir well and bring the mixture to boil.
2. Simmer the syrup for 3 to 5 minutes or until slightly thick, then remove the pan from the heat, whisk in xanthan gum until well mixed and the mixture is thick and set aside until required.
3. Prepare pudding and for this, place avocado in a blender, add remaining ingredients for pudding and pulse for 1 to 2 minutes or until smooth.
4. Divide the pudding evenly between two ramekins and place them into the refrigerator for 1 hour or more until chilled.
5. Then drizzle with prepared syrup and serve.

Nutritional facts

Calories: 171; Fat: 12g; Saturated fat: 7.3g; Net Carbohydrate: 1.7g; Protein: 1.1g; Fiber: 0.2g;

Chocolate Mousse

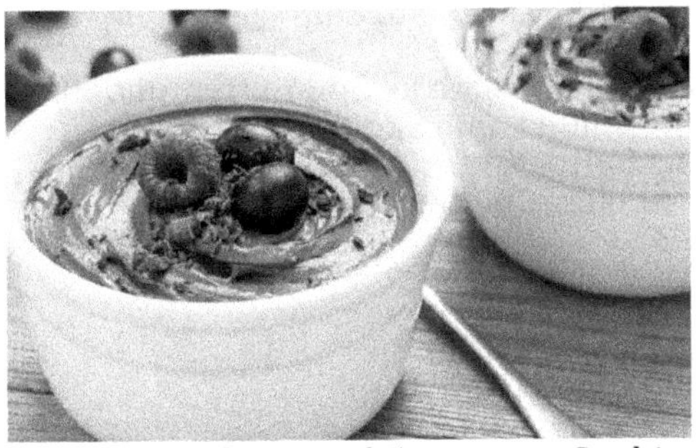

Prep time: 1 hour and 5 minutes, Cooking time: 0 minutes, Servings: 2

Ingredients

- Cream cheese, softened - 3 oz
- Vanilla extract, unsweetened - 1 tsp
- Heavy cream - ½ cup
- Salt - 1/16 tsp
- Swerve sweetener - ¼ cup
- Cocoa powder - 2 tbsp

Instructions

1. Place cream cheese in a bowl and beat using a stand mixer for 2 to 3 minutes at high speed or until fluffy.
2. Beat in vanilla and cream at low speed until combined and then beat in other ingredients until well incorporated.
3. Divide mousse evenly between two bowls and let refrigerate for 1 hour until chilled and then serve.

Nutritional facts

Calories: 373; Fat: 37.6g; Saturated fat: 23g; Net Carbohydrate: 5.3g; Protein: 5.4g; Fiber: 1.6g;

Meal Plan

Day1
Breakfast: Coconut Porridge
Lunch: Chicken Philly Cheesesteak Casserole
Dinner: Red Pesto Pork Chops
Dessert: Dark Chocolate Covered Walnuts
Day 2
Breakfast: Cinnamon Almond Butter Shake
Lunch: Fried Salmon with Green Beans
Dinner: Bacon-Wrapped Meatloaf
Dessert: Chocolate Gelato
Day 3
Breakfast: Cheese Crusted Omelet
Lunch: Turkey Soup
Dinner: Garlic Butter Steak
Dessert: Peanut Butter Cups
Day 4
Breakfast: French Pancakes
Lunch: BBQ Ribs
Dinner: Fish Fingers with Mayo Dip
Dessert: Lime Pudding
Day 5
Breakfast: Cauliflower Hash Browns
Lunch: Buffalo drumsticks
Dinner: Cajun Spiced Crab Casserole
Dessert: Chocolate Mug Cake
Day 6
Breakfast: Spinach and Avocado Smoothie
Lunch: Pork Carnitas
Dinner: Cashew Chicken
Dessert: Lemon Curd
Day 7
Breakfast: Chia Pudding
Lunch: Sesame Salmon with Thai Curry Cabbage
Dinner: Baked Salmon with Pesto
Dessert: Vanilla Ice Cream
Day 8
Breakfast: Beetroot Shake
Lunch: Butter Chicken
Dinner: Mozzarella Chicken
Dessert: Chocolate Gelato
Day 9
Breakfast: Mexican Scrambled Eggs
Lunch: Caesar salad
Dinner: Turkey with Cream-Cheese Sauce
Dessert: Dark Chocolate Covered Walnuts
Day 10
Breakfast: Green Breakfast Smoothie
Lunch: Salmon Meatballs
Dinner: Fried Salmon with Green Beans
Dessert: Lemon Curd
Day 11
Breakfast: Cheesy Bacon Cornbread Waffles
Lunch: Garlic Chicken
Dinner: Cuban Roast Pork
Dessert: Mint Chocolate Chip Ice Cream
Day 12
Breakfast: Chocolate Peanut Butter Smoothie
Lunch: Lemon Lamb Skewers
Dinner: Butter Cod
Dessert: Lime Pudding
Day 13
Breakfast: Frittata Muffin Cups
Lunch: Stuffed Zucchini Boats
Dinner: Garlic Scallops
Dessert: Vanilla Ice Cream
Day 14
Breakfast: Cinnamon Almond Butter Shake
Lunch: Shrimp Salad
Dinner: Lamb Chops with Herb Butter
Dessert: Chocolate Coconut Cups
Day 15
Breakfast: Frittata with Spinach
Lunch: Tuna Stuffed Tomatoes
Dinner: Turkey Soup
Dessert: Chocolate Mug Cake
Day 16
Breakfast: French toast
Lunch: Grilled Fish with Zucchini and Pesto
Dinner: Loaded Cauliflower
Dessert: Mint Chocolate Chip Ice Cream
Day 17
Breakfast: Chia Pudding
Lunch: Hamburger
Dinner: Cajun Spiced Crab Casserole
Dessert: Dark Chocolate Covered Walnuts
Day 18
Breakfast: Cauliflower Hash Browns
Lunch: Garlic Butter Salmon
Dinner: Rotisserie Chicken with Béarnaise Sauce
Dessert: Chocolate Gelato
Day 19
Breakfast: Cinnamon Almond Butter Shake
Lunch: Lamb Sliders
Dinner: Pork Carnitas
Dessert: Peanut Butter Cups
Day 20
Breakfast: Mexican Scrambled Eggs
Lunch: Cream Cheese Stuffed Peppers
Dinner: Bacon-Wrapped Meatloaf
Dessert: Vanilla Ice Cream
Day 21
Breakfast: Green Breakfast Smoothie
Lunch: Sesame Salmon with Bok Choy
Dinner: Mozzarella Chicken
Dessert: Chocolate Mousse

CPSIA information can be obtained
at www.ICGtesting.com
Printed in the USA
BVHW091104281021
620172BV00003B/195

9 781649 849854